'Faye Horsley presents a nuanced and richly informed perspective on fire, locating it within a broadly interdisciplinary account of human interactions with fire across time and cultures. Drawing on diverse sources, she compellingly argues that fire use in contemporary societies is best conceptualized as a continuum, and that a holistic approach is needed if we are to accurately assess and treat those who have used fire in a criminalised manner, or are on a path towards doing so. Accessibly written, this book will be of value to clinicians, jurists, and researchers alike; indeed, anyone who has been intrigued by fire and fire use will find their curiosity kindled.'

—**Daniel M. T. Fessler,**
University of California, Los Angeles

'*New Perspectives on Arson and Firesetting* provides a well-informed argument that many benefits will flow from.'

—**Richard Wrangham,**
author of Catching Fire *(New York: Basic Books, 2009)*

'This is a well-crafted book that will engage academic and lay inquisitive readers. It integrates theory along with careful consideration of pre-existing literature. It presents a new model to conceptualise firesetting, which applies a continuum approach as a helpful alternative to dichotomy. Consequently, I warmly recommend this valuable text.'

—**Jane L. Ireland,**
University of Central Lancashire, UK

'Horsley's accessible writing style, her practitioner and academic "voice", and the interdisciplinary approach she takes when unpicking the complex and fascinating relationship human beings have with fire is a welcome addition to the field. By shifting the traditional focus of firesetting research and practice away from the misuse of fire, and towards a wider notion of all fire use as a continuum of behaviour, Horsley provides a richer lens with which to think about children, teenagers and adults who set fires. With implications for research, assessment and practice, this book is an important addition in the armoury of those tasked with preventing and responding to fires.'

—**Joanna Foster,**
author and Managing Director of Fabtic, specialising in child-set fires

'This book is an excellent resource for practitioners and students alike in respect of a contemporary approach to firesetting and fire use. Risk assessment and treatment are considered, informed by theory but also from a practical perspective. This will help readers apply the useful recommendations for broad analysis of a person's relationship with fire, rather than only focusing on the firesetting that forms their offending behaviour. Firesetting requires careful analysis at an individual level; this book is an essential read that will certainly inform clinical practice and research in the future.'

—**Dr Ruth J. Tully,**
Consultant Forensic Psychologist and Clinical Lead at
Tully Forensic Psychology, UK

'This is a fascinating and authoritative book, taking an original look at fire and our relationship with it in order to raise serious questions about how we understand arson and "arsonists". In providing an in-depth exploration of the way humans in general understand and use fire, Dr Horsley has opened up an area of inquiry which has been significantly neglected, and offers us exciting and important insights, drawing out important connections between the ways we relate to fire in its conventional uses; unusual and symbolic fire practices; and the criminalisation of some forms of firesetting. The book also introduces an original and persuasive theory of fire use which represents a major original contribution to our knowledge and understanding of this fascinating subject.'

—**Professor Roger Smith,**
Durham University, UK

'*New Perspectives on Arson and Firesetting* is an exciting and innovative book that challenges traditional understandings of arson and firesetting, prompting us to think instead about a continuum of fire use. Dr Horsley pushes the boundaries of what we think we understand about fire use, through analysis of new evidence combined with clinical experience.'

—**Professor Laura Caulfield,**
University of Wolverhampton, UK

New Perspectives on Arson and Firesetting

New Perspectives on Arson and Firesetting: The Human-Fire Relationship is the first forensic text to move away from a sole focus on anti-social firesetting. The author presents a broader investigation of the role of fire in human life with a view to informing research and practice.

This book examines the evolutionary, psychological and social significance of fire. Drawing on interdisciplinary literature and original research data, it challenges the existing understanding of arson and firesetting. A new concept – fire use – is introduced, which is conceptualised as sitting on a continuum from non-criminalised to criminalised behaviour. The author combines her experience as a practitioner forensic psychologist with her own research to consider the practical application of an alternative perspective. This includes a particular focus on the assessment and treatment of firesetters and a call for a socially informed approach to prevention.

The forensic scope, applied focus, and emphasis on the importance of inter-disciplinary research and practice makes *New Perspectives on Arson and Firesetting* essential reading for students in fields such as anthropology, sociology, criminology, and psychology, as well as interdisciplinary scholars, forensic practitioners, and allied professionals.

The author is donating her royalties in full to Pancreatic Cancer UK.

Dr Faye K. Horsley is a lecturer in forensic psychology at Newcastle University. She is also a registered practitioner psychologist with over 16 years of experience working in prison and secure hospital settings.

New Frontiers in Forensic Psychology

Series Editors

Graham Towl is Professor of Forensic Psychology at Durham University and was formerly Chief Psychologist at the Ministry of Justice, UK. He is the recipient of the British Psychological Society Award for Distinguished Contributions to Professional Practice.

Tammi Walker is Principal of St Cuthbert's Society and Professor of Forensic Psychology at Durham University. She is a Chartered Psychologist and Fellow of the British Psychological Society, a Senior Fellow with Advance HE and a mental health nurse by clinical background.

New Frontiers in Forensic Psychology is a new series of forensic psychology books, which brings together the most contemporary research in core and emerging topics in the field, providing a comprehensive review of new areas of investigation in forensic psychology, and new perspectives on existing topics of enquiry. The series includes original volumes in which the authors are encouraged to explores unchartered territory, make cross-disciplinary evaluations, and where possible break new ground. The series is an essential resource for senior undergraduates, postgraduates, researchers and practitioners across forensic psychology, criminology and social policy.

Understanding Psychopathy
The Biopsychosocial Perspective
Nicholas Thomson

Child to Parent Aggression and Violence
A Guidebook for Parents and Practitioners
Hue San Kuay and Graham Towl

New Perspectives on Arson and Firesetting
The Human-Fire Relationship
Faye K. Horsley

For a complete list of all books in this series, please visit the series page at: https://www.routledge.com/New-Frontiers-in-Forensic-Psychology/book-series/NFFP

New Perspectives on Arson and Firesetting

The Human-Fire Relationship

FAYE K. HORSLEY

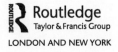

Routledge
Taylor & Francis Group

LONDON AND NEW YORK

First published 2022
by Routledge
2 Park Square, Milton Park, Abingdon, Oxon OX14 4RN

and by Routledge
605 Third Avenue, New York, NY 10158

Routledge is an imprint of the Taylor & Francis Group, an informa business

British Library Cataloguing-in-Publication Data
A catalogue record for this book is available from the British Library

Library of Congress Cataloging-in-Publication Data
A catalog record has been requested for this book

ISBN: 978-0-367-40710-0 (hbk)
ISBN: 978-0-367-40709-4 (pbk)
ISBN: 978-0-367-80864-8 (ebk)

DOI: 10.4324/9780367808648

Typeset in Avenir and Dante
by KnowledgeWorks Global Ltd.

FOR DAD, MUM AND LEE – THANK YOU.

AND FOR MY ABSENT LOVED ONES WHO
WILL NEVER GET TO READ THIS BUT WHOSE
MEMORY WILL FOREVER BURN BRIGHT.

Contents

List of figures and tables		xi
Series foreword		xii
Foreword		xiv
Preface		xvii

1 Introduction 1

Overview 1
Terms 1
The challenges 2
Progress 3

2 The significance of fire 6

Overview 6
The discovery of fire 7
Psychological aspects of fire 13
Fire play 16
Summary 19

3 The misuse of fire 20

Overview 20
Psychological research into arson and firesetting 22
A focus on risk 33
Implications 33
Summary 34

4   Understanding fire use   35

     Overview 35
     A meaningful dichotomy? 35
     Non-criminalised and criminalised fire use 38
     The Continuum of Fire Use (CoFU) 39
     Summary 42

5   A preliminary theory of fire use   43

     Overview 43
     Methodology 43
     Findings: the Continuum of Fire Use Theory (CoFUT) 45
     Application 58
     Evaluation and future directions 61
     Summary 62

6   Assessing people who set fires: A holistic approach   63

     Overview 63
     Forensic assessment 63
     Predisposing factors 64
     Precipitating factors and the offence analysis 71
     Risk monitoring and management 73
     Summary 75

7   Treatment and intervention with people who set fires   77

     Overview 77
     The CoFU 78
     The CoFUT 79
     Early intervention 85
     Summary 90

8   Conclusion   91

     Overview 91
     A holistic conceptualisation of fire use 92
     The social construction of fire 93
     Applications 94
     Thinking outside the box 95
     Future directions 97
     Summary 98

     References   *99*
     Index   *110*

List of figures and tables

Figures

2.1	The three polarities	19
4.1	The Continuum of Fire Use (CoFU)	40
5.1	Diagrammatic representation of the CoFUT	46
6.1	An extract from the FUM	67
6.2	The three polarities	69
6.3	The stage model of fire use	72

Tables

6.1	Fire Use Process Questions	73
7.1	Fire messaging	88

Series foreword

We warmly welcome this, first, book authored by Dr Faye Horsley entitled *New Perspectives on Arson and Firesetting: The Human-Fire Relationship* for our New Frontiers in Forensic Practice series. We publish two types of authored books; those with something different and innovative to say about existing forensic psychological practice, and new areas of forensic psychology. This original contribution to the field of firesetting from Dr Horsley falls in the former category revealing the limits of existing forensic psychological approaches to firesetting, whilst outlining her new model.

Dr Horsley's book takes an original exploration of firesetting and its interaction across time and culture among humans on an individual level. She moves away from only focusing on arson and firesetting as an 'offending behaviour' and calls for a more holistic approach to understanding this complex area. Through the presentation of data collected between 2014 and 2019 for her doctoral research she puts forward the idea that fire-related behaviour should be considered on a continuum - the Continuum of Fire Use Theory (CoFUT).

Dr Horsley's CoFU theory views fire *use* as a *process*, comprising a number of stages that moves from non-criminalised to criminalised fire use. Her novel approach, and, to our knowledge, the first ever theory of fire *use*, comprises of three themes, namely: Transient Emotional States, Sense of Self and Psychological Wellbeing. She argues that it is also equally important to consider the social construction of fire. This concept includes interrelated factors such as religion, culture, ethnicity, social norms and legislative frameworks. Dr Horsley maintains that understanding the evolutionary role of fire is of central importance because it has shaped the way we have come to view fire today and, indeed, the way we interact with it as a society. Dr Horsley's work sits in marked contrast with narrow conceptualisations of arson.

New Perspectives on Arson and Firesetting is a multi-disciplinary approach that is both a conceptual framework, i.e., a way of thinking about fire use, and also a practical tool for clinicians working with fire setters in the criminal justice and health care systems. Dr Horsley calls for forensic practitioners and researchers exploring and attempting to understand and reduce firesetting to 'think outside of the box'. The CoFUT re-conceptualises fire use and promotes a change in direction in forensic psychological practice in this area.

New Frontiers in Forensic Psychology brings together the most contemporary research in core and emerging topics in the field, providing a comprehensive review of new areas of investigation in forensic psychology and new perspectives on existing topics of enquiry.

The series includes original volumes in which the authors are encouraged to explore unchartered territory, make cross-disciplinary evaluations and, where possible, break new ground. Dr Horsley has certainly risen to that task and we believe that this book will be of wide interest both within and beyond the forensic psychological domain. The comments of international cross disciplinary reviewers attest to this.

The series is an essential resource for senior undergraduates, postgraduates, researchers and practitioners across forensic psychology, criminology and social policy.

Professor Tammi Walker and Professor Graham Towl
Series Editors
Department of Psychology, Durham University

Foreword

Dr Katarina Fritzon

I was delighted to be asked to write the foreword to this book, not least because although the literature on firesetting has been growing steadily over the last two decades, it is still heavily dominated by quantitative research. This book takes a different perspective, drawing on interdisciplinary literature to emphasise and illuminate the concept of fire *use* as a broader term than firesetting. It is therefore the first book to explore the idea of fire use as a continuum rather than attempting to dichotomise firesetters and non-firesetters. Before examining the detail of each of the chapters, I would like to make a few comments about the book as a whole. One of the most obvious aspects of the book, which readers will immediately notice, is that it is written in a way that is very engaging. Not only is the literature that is included very diverse, it is interwoven with quotes and examples from Dr Horsley's own (predominantly) qualitative research and there is a conversational tone which means that the book will appeal to academic and non-academic audiences alike. Secondly, despite its length, its coverage is very comprehensive. While not all existing research is summarised in depth, the most relevant is at least cited, so that the interested reader can explore further the aspects that are not described in detail within these pages. Lastly, the chapter that describes Dr Horsley's own qualitative research with illustrative quotes from real-life case examples marks this books' extension and advancement of knowledge in what is still very much an emerging field, particularly when it comes to risk assessment and management with those who have set fires.

Chapter 1 begins with a quote by anthroplogist Daniel Fessler, and this sets the scene for the broad range of literature that Dr Horsley draws on to synthesise her core themes of the book; the universal nature of fire across cultures and contexts; the synchronicity between the use and misuse of fire, and the usefulness of the conceptualisation of firesetting as a process rather than an event.

Chapter 2 considers the relationship between people and fire from historical, evolutionary and social perspectives, and draws on anthropological literature to argue that the central importance of fire in the progression of man's evolution[1] undoubtedly undoubtedly lies behind its continual and universal fascination. In discussing competing theories of how man came to harness fire, Dr Horsley intriguingly draws parallels with her own research, using quotes from her interview participants to illustrate the importance of both vicarious and 'hands on' learning of the many ways in which fires can be used and controlled by humans. In one of the more fascinating insights of this chapter, Dr Horsley suggests that in primitive communities where the functional properties and uses of fire are more observable, there may be an overt or covert prohibition against the *misuse* or frivolous use of fire (Fessler, 2006).

Chapter 3 then focuses on the misuse of fire more specifically, and summarises the psychological literature relating to fire risk assessment, characteristics of those who misuse fires, and firesetting/ arson typologies.

Chapter 4 begins to outline in depth the main thesis of the book, which is the false dichotomy between fire use and misuse. Referencing legal and criminological scholars on the often vexing delineation of what is legally, morally and socially acceptable, Dr Horsley once again highlights the particular challenge of fire use which in itself is not only functional but essential to human survival. Dr Horsley also parallels this point to that of positive psychology and the increasing emphasis on strengths alongside needs in the risk management literature within forensic psychology.

Chapter 5 is a summary of Dr Horsley's own qualitative research, in which she presents the Continuum of Fire Use Theory (CoFUT), which is described as "the psychology of the human-fire relationship as a whole, rather than solely a firesetting offence". Key themes representing the positive and negative impacts of fire, and highlighting the immediate gratification, Sense of Self and psychological wellbeing functions of fire use are illustrated through case examples and quotes.

Chapter 6 then applies the findings of this research to suggest an alternative approach to risk assessment through a case formulation approach, and the application of a Fire Use Matrix, which emphasises the motivation and target of the fire act (cf. Canter & Fritzon, 1998). The Fire Use Matrix is presented as a tool with potential for clinical use which requires research validation in order to determine its predictive utility. In developing a model of the stages of fire

---

1 For example, *the cooking of food expanded the range of food that could be consumed, leading to increased cognitive capacity (Wrangham, 2010).*

use, Dr Horsley also suggests that clinicians pay attention to the Instigation, Planning, Ignition, Active and Aftermath phases of the offence process; as well as examples of risk paralleling behaviour which may be informative in assessing and managing ongoing risk within institutional settings.

Chapter 7 deals with the application of the CoFUT to intervention, arguing for both psychological and sociological approaches including early intervention targeting the themes of *Transient Emotional States*, *Sense of Self*, and *Psychological Wellbeing*. In this chapter, Dr Horsley proposes that fire education programmes should emphasise the functional aspects of fire in order to perhaps reduce its more alluring appeal as a source of risk-taking and excitement.

In Chapter 8, Dr Horsley summarises the main themes of the book; the holistic conceptualisation of fire encompassing the Continuum of Fire Use and recognising the importance of themes of Transient Emotional State, Sense of Self and Psychological Wellbeing. Dr Horsley suggests a number of areas for future research, to further examine and validate aspects of her theory, and its applicability to assessment and intervention with individuals who use fire.

In examining fire use through the lens of multidisciplinary perspectives, Dr Horsley has expanded our ideas and themes about fire beyond the dichotomised and risk focused view of most forensic psychology firesetting research to date. The utility of socio-cultural and narrative based early intervention to prevent fire use from being glamourised or glorified remains to be tested, but researchers and practitioners alike will find much to inspire their thinking around fire within the pages of this book.

Preface

Before we begin, it is important to place this book, and why I am writing it, into context. I have been fortunate in my career so far to find the ideal balance of working as a practitioner forensic psychologist, as well as having the opportunity to teach the next generation of psychologists and to conduct research at Newcastle University. The content of this book marks the intersection of my professional experiences. It was through my practitioner life, working in prisons and secure hospital settings, where my interest in the psychology of firesetting first emerged. I have discovered through years of working clinically with people who set fires that they are complex, diverse and, at times, misunderstood. The psychological understanding of firesetting is nowhere near as well developed as that into some other types of offences (Gannon & Pina, 2010, p. 2; Doley, Dickens, & Gannon, 2016) and, even though the situation is improving, there are still areas which are yet to be explored (Butler & Gannon, 2020). My impression is, that for some, (practitioners and students alike) firesetting is just not viewed as psychologically interesting unlike offences such as homicide or sexual assault. Indeed, in my lecturer role, I find myself trying to 'sell' the topic to my students, many of whom might initially prefer to study sexual murder, serial killers or psychopathy to name but a few. Despite the initial ambivalence however, I have repeatedly found that once students and practitioners are introduced to the psychology of firesetting, the complex nature of this behaviour becomes clear. I hope that I can inspire you, as the reader of this book, to learn about the topic with the same degree of interest and open-mindedness. Let me start by explaining how I got here.

For 11 years I worked, full-time, as a forensic psychologist; first as a trainee and later as a qualified practitioner. My experience includes working in forensic hospitals and prisons ranging from high to low security both with men, women and young people in the public and private sector. In my various roles I have worked therapeutically with those convicted of crimes, in addition to conducting assessments of risk and need. Alongside my role as lecturer at Newcastle University, I continue to work as a forensic psychologist, mostly within the context of conducting assessments with people convicted of crime.

When working with forensic service users there are typically a range of assessment tools and treatment options at practitioners' disposal. However, I have found this not to be the case for firesetters, as I will expand upon in the next chapter. This likely reflects the aforementioned sparsity of firesetting research (until relatively recently at least) when compared to other types of crime. Observing the lack of specialist tools and treatments led me to question why there are so many gaps in our knowledge of how to work with those who set fires and so I began my research journey through embarking on a part-time Ph.D. in 2014. My research spanned four years and during this time I gave a number of conference presentations and public talks which represented a novel take on firesetting or, as I prefer to term it, fire *use*. I submitted the thesis to Durham University in December 2019. My thesis became publicly accessible in April 2020 and I finally graduated in August 2020, albeit under the cloud of a global pandemic.

This book draws on my doctoral research, alongside my practitioner experience. At the point of submission in December 2019 and its online publication in April 2020, my thesis represented a new way of thinking about how people interact with fire. In this book I hope to demonstrate that there is more than meets the eye to the understanding of firesetting or arson as it is referred to in the existing literature. I will argue that we should apply a much wider lens to the way we look at firesetting in order to understand the *relationship* humans have formed with fire over millions of years. Looking solely at firesetting as a criminal behaviour is, in my view, only part of the story. There are many benefits of interacting with fire and many positive uses which are yet to be explored within the psychological literature. I can think of no better way to start this book than with this illuminating quote from one of my research participants, George[2]: *"fire underpins so much of who we are, and what we do, and our history, and our culture, in ways that we haven't even scratched the surface of yet"*.

---

2 All participant names are pseudonyms in order to protect their identity.

Introduction 1

Overview

Although Fessler's position, elucidated in the following quote, dates back to 2006, I argue that it still stands true today: "We know little about the psychology of fire [and] fire learning... it is high time that we knew more" (2006, p. 448). Existing psychological research, which is almost solely focussed on the *misuse* of fire, only tells part of the story, and therefore, the psychological literature base is arguably a little one-sided. That being said, in the past decade, there has been significant progress in the psychological study of firesetting, which has made a substantial contribution to how forensic practitioners work with those convicted of firesetting offences. This progress is outlined below and referred to, in detail, in Chapter 3. First of all, this chapter will consider some of the key challenges in working with, and researching, people who set fires. As a starting point, it is prudent to clarify what terms I will be using in this book.

Terms

Psychological literature addressing the misuse of fire most commonly refers to either arson or firesetting. The former is a legal term (Daykin & Hamilton, 2012), whereas the latter constitutes "all deliberate acts of setting fire that are not recreational in nature" (Gannon & Barrowcliffe, 2012; p. 2). Unhelpfully, these terms are often used interchangeably (Horsley, 2020, 2021). In this book, I will refer to firesetting because this is more encompassing. However, where I am discussing literature which specifically refers to arson or arsonists, I will use

DOI: 10.4324/9780367808648-1

the same. There will therefore inevitably be some interchangeability of terms within this book which reflects the nature of the literature to date.

It is important to note in this introductory chapter that I will be arguing for a broader conceptualisation of human interaction with fire. I suggest that the term *fire use* better encompasses our complex relationship with fire and also reflects the notion that not all fire-related behaviour is reckless and illegal. Some of the challenges involved in the study of firesetting, and indeed, fire use will now be considered.

The challenges

One of the greatest challenges to understanding firesetting is rooted in the elusive and unpredictable nature of fire itself. Brett (2004) alludes to this in saying: "the initial intent of the firesetter does not always equate to the outcome...it is an adage among firefighters that a big fire is just a small fire that hasn't been controlled" (p. 419). Fire can be very difficult to control, even for professionals who have access to specialist equipment. In practice, this means that whilst someone who sets a fire might report only having intended to cause minimal damage to a property, the actual damage was much more catastrophic. In other words, their motivation (or, at least, that which they verbalise) does not necessarily equate to the outcome.

Another challenge in seeking to understand firesetting is the lack of research evidence. The work of practitioner psychologists and allied forensic and mental health practitioners should be evidence-based, meaning that we rely on good quality, contemporary research and theory to guide our practice. Problematically, however, the firesetting literature base is relatively sparse when compared to other offence types (Sambrooks and Tyler, 2019). For example, until 2012, there were only two multi-factorial theories of arson, namely the functional analysis model (Jackson, Hope & Glass, 1987) and the dynamic behaviour model (Fineman, 1995). Historically, research in this area is arguably flawed owing to the use of small and/or highly-specialist participant samples (for examples see Hurley & Monahan, 1969; Rice & Harris, 1991; Ritchie & Huff, 1999). The existing forensic psychological literature is considered in more detail in Chapter 3, but it is important to be aware of the notable gaps at this stage.

The relative dearth of firesetting literature means that, currently, there are no existing risk assessment tools specifically designed for people who set fires (Watt & Ong, 2016), nor are there any fully accredited treatment programmes (Palmer et al., 2007; Bell, 2016; Tyler, Gannon, Lockerbie & Ó Ciardha, 2018). In fact, a 'one size fits all' approach has generally been adopted with those who set fires (Horsley, 2020, p. 2). In other words, for decades there was an assumption that people who set fires should be dealt with, from an assessment and rehabilitative perspective, using the same approaches employed for other offences (i.e. violence and sexual violence).

Thankfully, this viewpoint is beginning to change (see Tyler et al., 2018) as we learn more about people who set fires and progress is made in empirical research. For example, through research designed to pinpoint a series of predictors for different types of crime, Edwards and Grace conclude that "the act of arson is different to both violent and non-violent offending" (2014, p. 226), which suggests that the 'one size fits all' approach is potentially insufficient.

Progress

The past decade has seen significant advances in the psychological understanding of firesetting. Researchers at the University of Kent's Centre of Research and Education in Forensic Psychology (CORE-FP) and colleagues have published widely on the topic which has improved what we know about firesetting (for examples, see Gannon et al., 2013; Ó Ciardha et al., 2015; Tyler, Gannon, Dickens & Lockerbie, 2015; Barrowcliffe, Tyler & Gannon, 2019; Butler & Gannon, 2020).

The work of the team at the CORE-FP has been highly influential. It includes the most up-to-date multi-factorial theory of adult firesetting *(the multi-trajectory theory of adult firesetting; M-TTAF;* Gannon, Ó Ciardha, Doley & Alleyne, 2012). The team is also behind the emergence of work using non-convicted samples (for example, Gannon & Barrowcliffe, 2012; Barrowcliffe & Gannon, 2015, 2016), with the premise being that many people who set fires remain un-apprehended and thus, it makes sense to study particular strands of the general population. Crucially, the work of the CORE-FP has practical application. The team has developed treatment programmes for those who set fires, such as the firesetter intervention programme for prisoners (FIPP; Gannon, 2013; as cited in Gannon et al., 2015) and a version for mentally disordered offenders (FIP-MO; Gannon & Lockerbie, 2011, 2012, 2014; as cited in Tyler et al., 2018), as well as a self-report measure (Ó Ciardha, Tyler & Gannon, 2015).

Whilst this progress is encouraging, it is important to note that treatment programmes such as the FIPP are designed for those who have already committed firesetting crimes or, at least, who are thought to be at particular risk of firesetting. In my view the same attention should be paid to the development and refinement of community-based 'early' interventions to help young people to form healthy relationships with fire. Currently, fire and rescue services (FRSs) are largely responsible for the delivery of such initiatives but there is little evidence of joined-up thinking on the matter from a national perspective

(Foster, 2020a). Additionally, their remit is mostly fire safety education (Foster, 2020a). In my view, this is at best insufficient and at worst inflammatory in that it could be increasing some young people's fascination with fire (returned to in more detail at various points in this book). There is, therefore, much progress still to be made in terms of the prevention of firesetting and a community-wide approach has a large part to play.

As mentioned earlier, the lack of impetus in developing clinical approaches specifically for firesetting until recently undoubtedly stemmed from a limited research base. Research by the CORE-FP team and others has improved the situation but there is still more work to do. Topics which I believe require more attention are elucidated in this book and introduced, briefly, below.

One problem, as we have already seen, is that existing psychological research focusses solely on the *misuse* of fire (either in the form of firesetting or the criminal offence of arson). I argue that this focus is too narrow and it means the psychology behind a myriad of ostensibly 'healthy' interactions with fire, such as the lighting of candles or enjoying log burners, has been neglected. Furthermore, so far fire-related behaviour has been dichotomised in the literature. More specifically, research participants have typically been categorised as either 'non-firesetters' or 'firesetters' (for examples see Ducat, McEwan & Ogloff, 2013; Gannon & Barrowcliffe, 2012; Barrowcliffe & Gannon, 2015, 2016). This approach is arguably an over-simplification of fire use, which is a very complex and heterogeneous construct. Also, the focus in the empirical literature on the act of *setting* or *lighting* fires has its limitations. I have already explained that I favour a broader term - fire use. Not only does this better capture a very diverse range of interactions with fire but it is also emblematic of what, I argue, should be thought of as a *process*, rather than a single event.

In my opinion there is also a risk of over-simplifying humans' interactions with fire through adopting a uni-disciplinary perspective. One of my core arguments is that we need to understand the human-fire *relationship*. To do this, we must fully appreciate how our species has come to use and view fire and how this has evolved over time. A historical appreciation of fire use is crucial because this likely forms the basis of how we view and interact with it today. This has support from the work of Presdee (2005) who writes about our complex relationship with fire from a social *and* historical perspective. In my view, psychology cannot possibly address these matters as a standalone discipline and so I am calling for an interdisciplinary approach. I hope to elucidate in this book that much can be learnt about human-fire use from anthropology and sociology and that drawing on published work from these disciplines, alongside psychology, could enhance our understanding of fire use. In particular, I assert that there needs to be more of an emphasis on the study of how fire is socially constructed. This is a multi-layered concept, comprising a myriad of interrelated factors such as religion, culture, ethnicity, social norms and legislative frameworks to name but a few. The role of fire in the evolution of our species is of central importance here because it has shaped the relationship we have formed with it. It is an exploration of this *relationship* which is, in my opinion, missing from existing psychological literature and which is the premise of this book.

The following two chapters represent a review of the interdisciplinary literature. Chapter 2 marks the starting point, namely, how our species first came to use fire and why it is so important in our lives today.

The significance of fire   **2**

Overview

As referred to in the previous chapter, there is much more to understand about the human relationship with fire than only how it is *mis*used. Fire plays a central role in our lives, and has done for millions of years. For these reasons, I argue that humans share a relationship with fire which has not yet been fully studied.

Knowledge of how our species first came to use fire is important if we are to understand how some have come to misuse it in the modern day. This is a common-sense principle which could be applied to any field of study. For example, contemporary scholars studying the Israeli – Palestinian conflict do not base their studies only on the nature of the conflict today. They examine the problems historically to trace them back to their roots, and they must study middle-eastern relations more broadly, taking account of manifold inter-relating factors such as religion, race, politics and economics. The same applies to the study of firesetting. I assert that we must adopt a perspective of fire use, which accounts for the history of our relationship with fire. This holistic approach has been lacking thus far in the forensic psychological literature.

This chapter draws on my previous work (Horsley, 2020, 2021) and considers fire's role in the evolution of our species, as well as how fire is socially con-structed, including the symbolism attached to it. All of these considerations are heavily intertwined with history and culture. Indeed, cultural considerations are a central theme in this book and, thus, it is important to outline what I am referring to in using this term. There is vast disparity in how culture has been defined but I favour a definition offered by Spencer-Oatey (2004), who suggests that culture is:

DOI: 10.4324/9780367808648-2

a fuzzy set of attitudes, beliefs, behavioural conventions, and basic assumptions and values that are shared by a group of people, and that influence each member's behaviour and each member's interpretations of the 'meaning' of other people's behaviour. (p. 3)

In accordance with the above definition, I consider that one's cultural background can be shaped by a multitude of factors including their country of origin, the country in which they were raised, their religious beliefs, the attitudes of their parents/care givers, race, ethnicity and life-long experiences.

This chapter will present an overview of the human-fire relationship from a number of different angles. It will explore humankind's symbolic, social and psychological connection with fire, alongside fire's biological and evolutionary significance (all of which interconnect). The latter is particularly important because some authors suggest that the human connection with fire is, at least, partly 'hard-wired' (for an example see Wrangham, 2010) which has implications for preventative and rehabilitative interventions targeting firesetting. Fire has also played a very important role in the geology of our planet (Pyne, 2019). Whilst not explicated in any great detail here, this is another point which must be acknowledged if we are to reach a more holistic understanding of the human-fire relationship.

As alluded to above, in order to explore the relationship we have formed with fire, we must trace this back to its inception, or perhaps more accurately, its inceptions.

The discovery of fire

The practical importance of fire to our species should not be underestimated. First and foremost, it is prudent to highlight what is surely the most irrefutable fact in relation to humans' reliance on fire – the existence of our sun. At the centre of our solar system, the sun's core temperature is about 27 million degrees Fahrenheit (NASA, 2017), which equates to roughly 15 million degrees Celsius. The sun's heat and light is the result of nuclear reactions at its core but at the most basic level we could think of it as a giant ball of fire; it is the lifeblood of our existence, without which there would be no life on Earth (NASA, 2017). As we move now to discuss how humans first came to experience fire and, later, to use it, the fact that the sun lies at the heart of our solar system and is the very root of our existence is a useful starting point.

Charles Darwin considered anthropogenic fire use[1] to be "...probably the greatest [discovery], excepting language, ever made by man" (Darwin 1871; cited in Wrangham, 2010, p. 10). Not only is this a vitally important skill, but it is also one which is unique to humans, therefore distinguishing us from other primates (Parker, 2015). Pyne (2019) notes that "since they first met, people and fire have rarely parted" (p. 119); however, exactly when that meeting first took place is difficult to establish (Gowlett & Wrangham, 2013). To explore this topic, it is necessary to look way beyond psychology, to the anthropological literature. Sandgathe (2017) convincingly argues that any attempt to pinpoint one moment in time when humans first came across fire is futile. He highlights a number of reasons for this, including the following: firstly, from an archaeological perspective it can be difficult to delineate evidence of naturally occurring fires (i.e. caused by lightening) from that of anthropogenic use. Secondly, Sandgathe notes that authors writing on the subject do not always distinguish between evidence of a single use of fire from the evidence of "habitual" use, i.e. when fire use became a regular feature in the lives of our ancestors (p. 360). Gowlett and Wrangham (2013) echo this sentiment by incorporating the term "continuous fire use"; they suggest that this dates back at least 1.5 million years ago (mya) but they describe many complexities in making sense of archaeological evidence on the matter.

In addition to the question of *when* mankind first discovered and came to use fire, the question of *how* has also received attention in the anthropological literature. Sandgathe argues that understanding how we came to interact with fire is best conceptualised as a process and he proposes a series of stages: (i) habituation to natural fire, for example, lightening; (ii) fire use; (iii) the maintenance of fire; and (iv) the manufacture of fire. Rationally, he suggests that there is clear "directionality" in these stages (p. 367), for instance, it makes sense to assume that our ancestors must first have learnt about the nature of fire and how to control it before being able to produce it. Sandgathe's ideas broadly support those of Fessler (2006) who argues that anthropogenic fire use comprises two facets: (a) the *control* of fire and (b) the *production* of fire. Fessler also alludes to a process conceptualisation rather than a one-off event. He surmises, logically, that the control of fire within the Homo genus must have emerged before the production of fire because our ancestors would have had to contend with naturally occurring fires such as those caused by lightning storms (p. 430). A stage conceptualisation of how humans came to use fire is also advocated by Pyne (1998) who highlights that our ancestors initially had to compete with lightening fire before capturing fire for their own use (p. 69).

According to Parker (2015) there are different theories regarding how our species developed pyrotechnic abilities. Wrangham (2009; as cited in Parker, 2015) suggests our ancestors may have first discovered fire serendipitously. More specifically, it is possible that whilst engaging in rock pounding to fashion tools for hunting, our ancestors noticed that sparks led to the occurrence of small fires. They may have actively begun to experiment with the flames, perhaps through playfully prodding one another with a burning branch. The instinct to move away from the flame, coupled with a fear response, was observed, and over time they came to adopt this as a means of warding off predators. Interestingly, Wrangham's scenario alludes to the notion of fire *play*, even over two mya. This behaviour is returned to later in this chapter.

An alternative to the "accidental" discovery of fire perspective has been proposed by Parker (2015, pp. 33–34). He asserts that our ancestors were forced to adapt to fire because its natural occurrence increased, across Africa, as a result of geographical and meteorological changes. Pyne (1998) agrees with the notion of adaptation over time, but he emphasises that our species adapted to the "fire regime" (p. 65), i.e. the *pattern* of natural fire and when it occurred rather than particular types of fire per se. He suggests that fire is just one of many disturbances, drought being another example, to which organisms have acclimatised over time.

A detailed appraisal of when and how our species first came to use fire is beyond the scope of this book, but it is important to be aware of the different debates on the topic. The central point here is the consensus that our ancestors somehow adapted to fire – this is a fundamental premise of this book because it is this, which is surely at the root of our relationship with fire today. Moreover, I suggest that this adaptation should be considered integral to the development of firesetting prevention strategies. There is little evidence of this currently, which may well be emblematic of a lack of interdisciplinary working.

Given that our specie's adaptation to fire is key to understanding the human-fire relationship, it is important to be clear on what is meant by the term. For the purpose of this book, we can loosely think of adaptation as an increasing familiarity with fire on the part of our ancestors, through which, eventually, they came to learn to produce and maintain it, meaning that it became central to their life. In order to do justice to this point, it is prudent to delve a little deeper to explore how our ancestors came to adapt to fire and what benefits it held for us as a species; there are many different viewpoints. Fire use might be a learned skill, which begins in childhood, as proposed by Fessler (2006). Interestingly, he notes parallels between the way in which children learn about predators and the acquisition of fire-management skills. Children, he says, are curious about the flammability of various materials and the consequences of manipulating or rearranging burning objects (p. 433). This is echoed by Jackson et al. (1987) who suggest that "fascination and experimentation with fire is a widespread feature of normal child development" (p. 176).

Children's learning about the utility and dangers of fire is not always a 'hands-on' process; Fessler argues that this would lead to frequent injuries on the part of the child. It seems feasible, therefore, that vicarious learning also takes place as children experience the hazards associated with fire from watching others and hearing their stories. From a psychological perspective, this is important because it highlights the significance of interpersonal relationships and the social environment in how our attitudes about fire have been shaped over time. This is supported by data from my research (Horsley, 2020), which is discussed in more detail in Chapter 5. I interviewed a number of fire users who made reference to the influence of others in how their fire narratives have developed. For example, Viv recalls her mother "nagging about fires in the past; like when you leave something in the oven and it's burning". Likewise, Tia's grandmother regularly "drilled" the dangers of fire into her and her siblings.

In summary, Fessler (2006) suggests we may have learnt to use fire; a view supported by Wrangham (2010). Importantly, Fessler also asserts that the control of fire carried many advantages for our ancestors – a point which is widely agreed upon. For example, it aided our ancestors in searching for food by enabling them to clear grassy landscapes, meaning that prey and food could be discovered more easily (Parker, 2015). Fire also served as a source of heat and light, which offered an antidote to cold and darkness and, in turn, this helped to keep predators at bay (Goudsblom, 1992; Clark & Harris, 1985), as well as extending the day (Lynn, 2014). Furthermore, fire enabled our ancestors to produce tools (Pyne, 1998; Fessler, 2006), which were essential for hunting and gathering food sources. In addition, it has been argued that our ancestors' engagement in fireside rituals fostered a meditative-like state which, in turn, was responsible for enhanced working memory capacity and, more broadly, contributed to a healthy mind (Rossano, 2007). Lastly, the relaxing properties of fire and, the physiological benefits of this, have also been discussed in anthropological literature (for example, see Lynn, 2014).

It is fair to say that there is a general consensus about the advantages of fire use for our species. However, there are some who extend this idea further by suggesting that fire has played a role in evolution by *natural selection* (for example, see Wrangham, 2010; Wrangham & Carmody, 2010; Wrangham, 2017). In other words, according to some, our species' ability to control and use fire led to physical changes over millions of years. These changes were advantageous, thus, aiding survival and were passed on (genetically) from generation to generation. According to this viewpoint, our species underwent physical changes *because* of our use of fire. Wrangham (2010) discusses many examples of these changes, one of which is the shrinking in size of our digestive system. This, he suggests, was a direct consequence of our ancestors' discovery of fire and their use of it to cook food. Cooking food means it is more easily digested and, hence, our digestive system became smaller and so our net energy gain from food became higher. Additionally, food was more tender and so less chewing was required (again, meaning a higher net energy gain). Furthermore, Wrangham suggests fire served a protective function by warding off prey, which enabled our ancestors to sleep soundly. Wrangham (2010) asserts that these benefits, which were all the result of using fire to cook food, led to an increase in cranial capacity, which is the root of the advanced cognitive ability of modern-day humans. Other benefits of cooking are cited in Goudsblom (1992), such as an increase in the range of foods which could be consumed and the reduction of disease. It is important to note that theories about the role of fire in evolution by natural selection have not gone uncontested, because there are debates about the extent to which they are supported by archaeological evidence (Parker, 2015, p. 32), but such a discussion is beyond the scope of this book.

Whether one accepts the argument about fire's role in natural selection or not, the important point for readers of this book is that we have come to be *reliant* on fire for a variety of reasons over millions of years and this stems back to our hunter-gatherer roots (Parker, 2015). In referring to the evolution of our species throughout this book, I use this term in its broadest sense, i.e. that fire has contributed to how we have changed over time, including physical, sociological and psychological changes. These fire-related changes are of central importance in understanding the reconceptualisation of arson which I am proposing. The fact that the human-fire relationship is complex, multi-faceted and dates back millions of years must be, in my view, front and centre in the understanding of arson/firesetting and in the work of forensic practitioners. Currently, whilst it is alluded to in the forensic psychological literature (for example, see Gannon et al., 2012), it has not been expanded upon.

The evidence that fire featured in our ancestors' lives is unequivocal. Indeed, Pyne (2016) notes that prior to the last century, fire was ubiquitous: "working fires cooked, warmed, enlightened, entertained, worshipped and transmuted dross substances and landscapes into usable goods and habitats…the first act of a day was to kindle a fire; the last act, to bank the coals; and in between, fire was a constant companion" (p. 1). Fire continues to be crucial for our survival today; however, we, in the developed western world, are less aware of it, which is a point argued by Pyne (2016). For example, although around 80% of the world's energy is still gleaned through the burning of fossil fuels (Nunez, 2019) when we turn on our gas cooker few of us would give much thought to this being a form of fire use. Likewise, by flicking a switch a large proportion of us in the UK have access to gas central heating which almost instantaneously warms the radiators in our home. However, in doing so, we need not be aware of the mechanisms behind the source of heat. Even if we consider the gradual move towards renewable energy sources, such as solar power, we return to the fundamental point that the sun is, itself, a form of fire on which we are entirely reliant.

I assert that in the Global North our dependence on fire for survival is generally now less overt. This is because our exposure to fire in its rawest form, the naked flame, has lessened greatly with the invention of technology. This is supported by the work of Gowlett (2016) who refers to "hidden fire" (p. 1) and Pyne (2016) who notes that the "interplay between people and flame" in industrialised city life has now ceased. Therefore, in the Global North, many of us take for granted the essential role that fire plays in life. Conversely, in certain countries and specific communities, fire is engaged with more overtly and is employed as a functional tool.

An example of the functional use of fire, which contrasts greatly with contemporary fire use in the UK, is provided by Fessler (2006). He observed a semi-traditional Bengkulu Malay fishing village on the west coast of Sumatra where fire is "routinely used as a tool" (p. 438). He notes that, here, children interact with fire from an early age, but there is very little fire play as we might observe in the developed world. In this community, Fessler found that from the age of around six children are assigned fire-related tasks, such as collecting material and, after a few years, they are tasked with cooking and tending to fires. Crucially, combining his own findings and those of the ethnographers whom he surveyed, Fessler hypothesises that in communities where a fire is used as a daily tool, it holds less entertainment value (p. 440). It is noteworthy that research by Murray, Fessler and Lupfer (2015) and Sherrell (2021) highlights that this is by no means a straightforward matter, which is returned to in Chapter 7.

Another example of functional fire use is described by Mistry et al. (2005) who studied the use of fire by indigenous peoples in the Cerrado (Savannas) of Brazil and found a broad range of motivations behind its use, including:

- The cultivation of land in order to clear and prepare it for farming;
- For hunting through attracting game;
- The harvesting of natural resources, for instance, fire stimulates the growth of certain fruits;
- Aesthetic reasons, such as keeping land clean and reducing vegetation to improve visibility;
- Protective functions, including the burning of land which might otherwise increase the chance of conflagrations later, such as the bush fires seen in Australia;
- To eliminate pests, such as snakes (pp. 371–372).

Interestingly, Mistry et al. (2005) observed a "very permissive attitude towards children playing with fire" amongst elders in their study (p. 375). They note regular instances where children would run around the village holding burning palm leaves, which was met with a lack of concern from their parents. Mistry et al. highlight that fire is an essential tool for the indigenous peoples they studied because their low income renders technological alternatives infeasible. Populations such as those studied by Mistry et al. (2005) and Fessler (2006) therefore perhaps better reflect the way our ancestors may have interacted with fire in that they, too, had no access to modern-day technology. These studies also point to cultural variation, not only in how fire is engaged with but also in how it is socially constructed, i.e. perceived by people. This is returned to below.

So far, our species' adaptation to fire has been discussed, along with its role as a functional and practical tool. The overtness of this reliance may differ across cultures (including different countries) depending on the relative accessibility of modern technology which, to some degree, masks the relevance of fire in its rawest form. Arguably, in the UK and other technologically advanced countries in the Global North, we have come to place more importance on our *psychological* and *social* connection with fire, rather than recognising it as something on which we physically depend. I suggest that understanding this shift in the use and social representations of fire is key to developing effective firesetting treatments/interventions in the UK.

Psychological aspects of fire

Fire undoubtedly carries a degree of importance from a psychological and sociological perspective. For example, Presdee (2005) explains that our emotions and fire are intertwined, and that fire plays an important role in human identity. Socially, if we consider our own lives, we can likely identify times where fire has featured as part of a social event, for example in the form of a barbeque or a communal bonfire, and we might reflect on how this impacted us psychologically. Indeed, Lynn (2014) notes that several scholars have written about the social connection associated with gathering around a fire. If we stop to consider it, we will find that fire, both in a physical and metaphorical sense, is truly omnipresent and that it is an integral part of the human psyche; some of the evidence for this idea is explored below.

Symbolism and fire

As previously discussed, we came to rely on fire over millions of years in a practical sense, but, at some point, we also came to attach symbolism to it. In other words, we came to see fire as having meaning beyond the fire itself. For example, research in the USA has highlighted how some people view it as having paranormal qualities, akin to alien visitation, reincarnation and astrology (Messer & Griggs, 1989). Further, Winder (2009) reminds us that fire represents "a beacon of hope, means of blessing, healing and protection" (p. 15) and Hardesty and Gayton (2002) discuss how it is conveyed as "stimulating, provocative, positive and powerful" in films, music, and literature (pp. 1–2). Similarly, fire features in our vernacular in ways we might not even be aware of, for instance, Pinsonneault (2002b) cites phrases such as "[putting up a] smoke screen" which relates to deceiving someone, to "walk on hot coals" in reference to proving one's loyalty, and "carrying a torch" which relates to one's attraction to another person (p. 27). In most, if not all cases, fire-related words are associated with power, danger, sexuality and mystery, which Pinsonneault aptly highlights might be sending worrisome signals to young children (p. 28) – this is returned to in Chapter 7.

For the participants in my qualitative study (Horsley, 2020; outlined in Chapter 5), symbolic representations of fire are just as important as its physical properties and this may well reflect people in the UK (where my research was based) more widely. The degree and nature of emphasis placed on the symbolic meaning of fire is likely to vary across different cultures (which, as referred to earlier, includes different countries, races, ethnicities and religions). I suggest that an insight into the symbolic representation of fire is integral to our comprehension of firesetting and the design of appropriate treatment/interventions. For example, if we identify problems in the messaging conveyed to young people about fire then this might enable us to seek to change this message – this is returned to in Chapter 7.

Symbolic references to fire are a historical phenomenon. They appear within Greek and Roman mythology, for example, Topp (1973) explains that in Greek mythology Hestia was the appointed Goddess of the hearth and that her fire was to be maintained as a place of worship and protection. Similarly, Zeus was the God of the sky to whom the sun belonged. Likewise, Pyne (2016) provides other examples of fire's omnipresence in mythology, for example, the rising of the Phoenix from the ashes (p. 2). The symbolic significance of fire features widely in religion. Indeed, Argyle (as cited in Winder, 2009) suggests that the earliest forms of religious worship were fire-related and Winder (2009) highlights its ongoing significance in religion today, with particular reference to Paganism and Wicca, where fires and candles are used in rituals throughout the year. Similarly, Pyne (2016) refers to religious representations of fire, in which for some "fire was a god" and for others "a manifestation of divine presence" (p. 2).

Although fire is a ubiquitous feature of many religions, the symbolism ascribed to it is diverse, multi-layered and complex. For example, in Catholicism, candles are used to convey one's devotion and reverence to God (Schoenstatt Scotland, 2015) and in Judaism, the eight candles of the Menorah are lit during Hanukkah in celebration of the victory of the Jews in recapturing Jerusalem from Syrian Greeks (BBC, 2009). It is not only in the form of candles where fire is used in religion. Winder (2009) refers to the burning of bodies in funeral pyres in Hinduism and Christianity, which is a symbolic act of "freeing the soul of the deceased" (p. 14). Further, in an ethnographic study of Holiness snake handlers in Southern Appalachia, Kane (1982) reports on the ritualistic handling of fire – curiously with no visible sign of injury – as a way of proving dedication to and faith in God, in addition to demonstrating the power of God (p. 375). Another example is cited in Danforth (1989) who writes of a Northern Greek ritual that involves fire walking, dating back to the 1920s. In this annual "ritual cycle" (p. 4) culminating on 21st May townsfolk dance and engage in fire walking in the belief that St Constantine will heal them of illness.

The ritualistic use of fire does not always have religious meaning (although arguably this could depend on how one defines religion). It is also used symbolically in ceremonies, celebrations and for entertainment (Presdee, 2005). Indeed, Presdee (2005) writes about fire's intriguing dualities, such as that of "destructiveness and creativity" (p. 74), which perhaps indicates why it is viewed as so exciting, intriguing and mesmerising.

Fire in celebrations and for entertainment

Fire has long been a feature of social interaction, which is epitomised in the fact that the Latin word for hearth is focus, leading Pyne (2019) to suggest that fire was traditionally the centre of every home (p. 103). Similarly, Goudsblom (1992) notes that fire has always been integral to group life because of the comfort and security it offers.

Indeed, fire plays a central role in group celebrations around the world. For example, Konvalinka et al. (2011) refer to an annual fire-walking ritual which takes place in a rural Spanish village to mark the summer solstice within a large amphitheatre. Once a large fire is reduced to ash, participants dance before walking across the hot coals, usually whilst carrying a relative on their back. Similarly, between 1st and 19th March each year, Valencia in Spain hosts the Fallas celebrations in which works of art are displayed in the city and then burnt, as a way of marking the beginning of spring (Visitvalencia.com, 2021). Winder (2009) also highlights the use of fire in the form of the Olympic torch which is revealed at the opening ceremony of each Olympic Games.

Another well-known example of the use of fire for celebratory purposes is The Burning Man Festival, held annually in the Nevadan Desert, USA. This is described as a festival of arts and creativity, with a carnival-type atmosphere and a spiritual, rather than religious tone (Gilmore, 2010). The culmination of the festival is the burning of a wooden figure, packed with explosives, which is 40 feet in height (Clipper, 2007; Gilmore, 2010). Finally, a world-renowned ritual dating back to the 1600s in England is that of 5th November; now commonly known as 'bonfire night'. This relates to the plot by Guy Fawkes and co-conspirators to commit treason by blowing up the houses of parliament with gunpowder (Sharpe, 2005). In the 1600s Londoners were encouraged to light bonfires to celebrate the uncovering of this plot. Nowadays in the UK, I assert that the entertainment value of fire, such as the lighting of bonfires and fireworks, supersedes the historical significance for many who engage in such celebrations. Therefore, the 5th November celebration in the UK is an example of where the underlying symbolism has waned and is not the primary motivation for the millions of people who celebrate with bonfires and fireworks nowadays (Sharpe, 2005).

As seen above, symbolic representations and celebratory uses of fire are manifold. I am suggesting that all of this is, or should be, of central importance for professionals working with people who set fires. This is important both in conducting assessments, for example, by seeking to understand what fire *means* to a particular service user and also in developing treatment and interventions.

The symbolism ascribed to fire, as well as celebratory uses, interconnect with another important consideration – the entertaining qualities of fire. In the existing academic literature the most commonly cited use of fire for what could constitute entertainment purposes is *fire play*, which is defined by Hall (2000) as "a fire deliberately set for no purpose, constructive or destructive, beyond the fire itself" (p. 1). In the following section, what is known about fire play is explored. A discussion on fire play appears at this point in the chapter because it leads us into the following chapter which addresses arson and firesetting. I suggest that fire play might mark an intersection between what is considered appropriate and acceptable use of fire (which I term non-criminalised fire use) and what is viewed as criminalised fire use (which includes arson and firesetting).

Fire play

As the indigenous research by Mistry et al. (2005) illuminated, what is considered as acceptable or unacceptable fire-related behaviour likely has cultural undertones. Mistry et al. referred to the lack of concern from the indigenous parents whose children played with burning palm tree leaves but the same behaviour might be perceived differently by many parents in the UK. Fire play is a highly complex concept because there are myriad of considerations, including how to define it and the many gradations of the behaviour.

Research in the USA has demonstrated that fire play is relatively common in children and that it can increase linearly with age up to a point (Grolnick, Cole, Laurenitis, & Schwartzman, 1990). However, whether such behaviour is considered "normal" in young people is open to debate (Fritzon, Dolan, Doley & McEwan, 2011, p. 395). Fessler (2006) asserts that fire play should not be considered harmless and that fire safety officers' concern with it is quite justified (p. 434).

Whilst research into the prevalence of fire play amongst children and adolescents has been conducted, the variability in the way the behaviour is defined means that exact prevalence rates are difficult to establish. Furthermore, a lot of this research originates from outside of the UK, meaning that generalisability could be a problem. That being said, studies based in western countries, such as the USA or Australia, are likely applicable here to some extent at least. There have been a number of studies into fire play. For example, Simonsen and Bullis (2001; as cited in Murray, Fessler & Lupfer, 2015) surveyed over 5,000 third to eighth-grade students in Oregon, USA. Forty-seven percent of respondents reported to have played with fire between the ages of 1 and 15. Interest in fire was reportedly high, as was the perceived entertainment value, for example, 23% of the sample started fires "for fun". In another study, with a sample of 138 young people "match-play", which included "playing with candles and striking matches" (p.21) was considered to be an acceptable form of behaviour, i.e. '*non*-firesetting' (Kolko & Kazdin, 1992). This study found that across three-time points in a one-year period, over 50% of participants had played with matches. Crucially, Kolko and Kazdin refer to the overlap between match play and firesetting, which supports my assertion that playing with fire could mark the intersection between non-criminalised and criminalised fire use. In a more recent study Perrin – Wallqvist and Norlander (2003) qualitatively investigated young men and women's interest in playing with fire in Sweden. In total, 70% of men and 44% of women admitted to playing with fire as children.

As referred to earlier, Fessler (2006) contrasts the way in which children in a semi-traditional Bengkulu Malay fishing village on the west coast of Sumatra interact with fire with those in contemporary societies. In the fishing community, fire is "routinely used as a tool" (p. 438) and children interact with it from an early age. In his observations, he notes very little fire play as we might observe in the developed world (p. 446). As referred to above, the key point here is that, according to Fessler, fire holds less entertainment value in communities where it is used as a tool (p. 440). Conversely, Fessler suggests that in the western world most children seldom have the opportunity to interact with fire because they are not frequently exposed to it. Therefore, adolescence may be the first opportunity to "experiment" (p. 438), which might be a form of rebellion, also referred to by Pinsonneault (2002b). Gannon et al. (2012) echo this sentiment by referring to the "forbidden" nature of fire in western culture which is why, here, children have less opportunity to learn about it (pp. 19–20) and, indeed, less exposure to it.

As epitomised by the work of Mistry et al. (2005) and Fessler (2006), a person's cultural background seems to be a likely determinant of how they interact with fire and what they consider to be fire play. In other words, the fire-related beliefs of people living in the UK where our reliance on fire is less overt may be quite different from those of people who routinely utilise fire (in its most primitive form) as a functional tool. Such a difference in 'fire narratives' has never been systematically explored; however, it seems plausible based on existing research findings. Pinsonneault (2002b) alludes to this in her appraisal of the relevance of fire at each developmental stage of childhood/adolescence. At the pre-school age she suggests that children may be confused about how to conceptualise fire in the absence of a "functional category" to place it in, for instance, "a thing to cook with" (p. 19). Essentially, then, whereas children in some cultures are readily able to categorise fire as a functional tool, children in western developed countries, such as the UK, might not automatically do so. It is possible, that this issue continues beyond pre-school age if a young person never comes to associate it with a purposeful activity such as cooking or heating.

Of central importance to this book is that such cultural variations are of relevance in understanding firesetting and, importantly, how to reduce it. I suggest that we might be able to learn from studying how young people in other cultures interact with fire to foster the same relationship, or at least the same fire-related beliefs, in young people in the UK. The lack of everyday exposure to the mundane and practical features of fire may be problematic in the UK. Furthermore, I suggest that fire is 'taboo' in this country which might, in some cases, actually serve to increase children's intrigue and might evoke a desire to rebel through playing with fire. I suggest that these points should lead us to question current practice in the UK – this is returned to in Chapter 7.

In this chapter, I have proposed that the degree of functionality of fire or at least the overtness of that functionality likely differs across different cultures. Some cultures around the world use fire very overtly as a tool by cooking over an open flame or using it to fertilise land, whereas others are probably less aware of its functional role because it is often masked by modern technologies such as central heating or electric ovens. Also discussed in this chapter is the idea that the level and nature of symbolism associated with fire may well be culture specific. Furthermore, in some cultures fire is arguably more taboo than in others. These considerations can be depicted by way of three polarities, which I propose could inform future thinking on, and research into, fire use (see Figure 2.1). I will refer to these polarities in more detail in Chapters 6 and 7. They relate to the way in which fire is *subjectively perceived* by people in a particular population i.e. – in other words, the way it is socially constructed and can be summarised as follows.

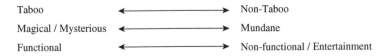

Taboo	Non-Taboo
Magical / Mysterious	Mundane
Functional	Non-functional / Entertainment

Figure 2.1 The three polarities.

Summary

In this chapter, interdisciplinary literature has been drawn upon in order to demonstrate the longevity and complexity of the human-fire relationship. It is an indisputable fact that humankind is entirely reliant on fire for survival and to find the evidence of this we need to look no further than the sun; the centre of our solar system. This exemplifies why, in my opinion, a focus only on the *mis*use of fire is too narrow. As demonstrated above, fire holds symbolic, social and psychological significance for humans, much of which is strongly influenced by cultural background. Furthermore, it has played an integral role in our past and evolution to an extent that some (for example, see Wrangham, 2010) even argue that it has contributed to evolution by natural selection. An appreciation of these points is crucial if we are to reach a fuller understanding of why and how people *mis*use fire; this is the focus of the next chapter.

Note

1 **Anthropogenic fire use:** The use of fire by humans.

The misuse of fire 3

Overview

Fire not only has empowering qualities but also a capacity for destruction (Winder, 2009; p. 11). This is referred to by Bachelard (1938/1964; as cited in Winder, 2009, p. 11) as fire's "opposing values of good and evil". The capacity of fire to do harm is summarised by participants in my own research (Horsley, 2020). For example, Sherry says: "it can kill people. Or leave them badly scarred. It can destroy families and friendships" and Tia speaks of fire's deceptive nature through personifying a candle flame: "it looks really innocent, doesn't it? It's really innocent on its little candle stick; all cute and smelling nice. But if it was knocked over it could just burn down a full house".

In the UK today it is clear that we are aware of the dangers of fire, as exemplified by stringent legislation aimed at promoting fire safety in England, such as the Regulatory Reform (Fire Safety) Order of 2005 and the Smoke and Carbon Monoxide Alarm Regulations of 2015. Although many fires are accidental, fire can also be used by people to deliberately harm and/or cause damage. This behaviour is usually referred to as arson or firesetting in the literature. In Chapter 1 the distinction between these two terms (the former being a legal term) was outlined, although they tend to be used interchangeably within the literature. Firesetting is a worldwide problem (Tyler, Gannon, Ó Ciardha, Ogloff & Stadolnik, 2019). According to official statistics for England in the year ending December 2020 the fire and rescue service (FRS) attended just over 65,000 deliberate fires with 37 fatalities and 940 non-fatal casualties reported (Home Office, 2020). It is the misuse of fire, which will be explored in this chapter building on my previous work (Horsley, 2020; 2021). In this chapter, there will be some

DOI: 10.4324/9780367808648-3

interchangeability in terms, namely, arson or firesetting, which reflects the existing literature.

The task of determining what, exactly, constitutes the misuse of fire, and to what extent, is not as straightforward as it may at first seem. How behaviour is defined will be explored in more detail in Chapter 4, but at this stage it is important to highlight that this is open to conjecture. One's own opinion on what is appropriate fire use is likely influenced by manifold factors, such as the way fire is constructed in their society and societal norms, cultural context and one's moral stance. It could also vary across time; the execution of those convicted of crimes by burning in England is one example. This practice was lawful in England until 5th June 1790 (Campbell, 1984). It was most often issued to women for a range of offences including petty treason, counterfeiting (Campbell, 1984) and theft (Reinhard, 1941). In addition, burning at the stake was, at one time, commonplace across the world for those suspected of witchcraft (Riddell, 1929; Reinhard, 1941). I suggest that whether one views this practice as an appropriate punishment or a barbaric act may reflect the passing of time. It might be that it was accepted as the norm in the past but the execution by burning in contemporary Britain would likely be viewed quite differently, at least by a significant portion of the population.

The existing psychological academic literature reflects the aforementioned variability in that there is a troublesome lack of consensus on what should be classed as non-firesetting or firesetting (for examples of different definitions, see Geller, 1992; Davis & Lauber, 1999; Doley, 2003; Vaughn et al., 2010). This lack of consensus has generally been air-brushed over and is seldom referred to directly within the literature, which is problematic. We surely cannot meaningfully interpret existing research findings about any human behaviour if we are unclear on the particulars of the behaviour of interest. For instance, where researchers have explored psychological differences between non-firesetters and firesetters, we can only be confident that these characteristics truly delineate the two groups if the behaviours are clearly demarcated. The lack of clarity in terms used within the literature should be borne in mind as the current state of play is addressed, below.

There are also other issues with the existing literature, meaning there are a number of unknowns with respect to firesetting. The unknowns which are most relevant to this book were reviewed in the introductory chapter and are briefly summarised again here. First, whilst we now know more about the psychology of arson and firesetting, we know very little about non-criminalised forms of fire use (such as those discussed in Chapter 2) from a psychological perspective. Secondly, I consider human interactions with fire to be a process rather than a one-off event and, thus, it would make sense to explore the stages of fire use, rather than solely focussing on the ignition of fire as most research has done (see Chapter 6 for more detail). Lastly, the non-firesetting/firesetting dichotomy might over-simplify a very complex and heterogeneous construct – this is expounded in Chapter 4. These methodological and conceptual issues will be returned to throughout this chapter as the existing forensic psychological literature is reviewed.

Psychological research into arson and firesetting

As discussed in Horsley (2021), research into criminalised fire use, in the form of arson and firesetting has prevailed within the psychological literature when compared to non-criminalised use. This research can be organised into three categories on the basis of the main focus of the work: (i) recidivism and dangerousness, (ii) characteristics of arsonists/firesetters, and (iii) the classification of arsonists/firesetters, including theoretical perspectives, each of which will be discussed in turn below. It is important to note that the categories outlined above are, by no means, mutually exclusive. For instance, studies which have addressed recidivism rates in a sample of arsonists/firesetters might also explore the characteristics of that group, when compared to those committing other crimes. I have chosen to present a review of the research using these sub-headings as a way of making sense of the existing literature base, which spans many decades. Before moving on to review the literature, however, it is useful to highlight certain caveats relating to the existing literature.

Caveats

Gender

First and foremost, arguably the most obvious issue with the literature in this field is that women who set fires have been neglected (Long, Fitzgerald & Hollin, 2015). This means that our understanding of men who set fires is much more comprehensive – an issue which is also true across the forensic psychology literature more broadly (Gannon, Tyler, Barnoux & Pina, 2012). But how different are men and women who set fires? If the differences are minimal then, perhaps, we can draw some assumptions about women on the basis of what we know of men.

Characteristics so far associated with women who set fires include child victimisation, mental disorder, relationship difficulties, poor interpersonal problem solving, mental health difficulties and emotional regulation issues (Gannon, 2010; Fritzon & Miller, 2016) but these are not necessarily specific to women.

Crucially, Gannon et al. (2012) note that very little research has systematically *compared* men and women who set fires; thus we really know very little about gender differences in firesetting – a point echoed by Fritzon and Miller (2016). From what we know so far there does appear to be, at least, some overlap between men and women, namely in socio-demographic features, developmental background, offence histories and motives (Gannon, 2010; Gannon et al., 2012). There is also an indication that women who light fires share much in common with women who commit other crimes (Fritzon & Miller, 2016).

In the following review of the literature, I have not sought to highlight the gender composition of the individual studies which are cited. Owing to the lack of definitive evidence at present doing so would risk complicating matters and could lead to a number of distracting tangents. Needless to say, however, there is a perceptible need for further research which not only includes women in the participant pool but also specifically compares women and men who set fires (Gannon et al., 2012). Furthermore, I would argue that there is now a need to look beyond the binary man/woman categorisation and to consider gender *identity* in relation to firesetting (and, for that matter, all crimes).

Forensic status

As referred to above, the majority of psychological empirical research on firesetting has focussed on arsonists, i.e. those convicted of an offence through the Criminal Justice System (CJS), whom either reside in prison or psychiatric hospitals (for examples, see Hurley & Monahan, 1969; Prins, Tennent & Trick, 1985; Jackson et al., 1987; Rix, 1994; Lindberg, Holi, Tani & Virkkunen, 2005). Daykin and Hamilton (2012) challenge the use of convicted samples and argue that poor detection rates for arson mean that this approach is "likely to be limited and speculative" (p. 11). A parallel can perhaps be drawn here with much of what we claim to know about those convicted of sexual crimes. Much of such work has been based on convicted samples, who are the overwhelming *minority* of people convicted of sexual offences (Towl, 2018). It could, therefore, be reasonably hypothesised that such samples are unrepresentative. Yet this is not always acknowledged in the sexual offending literature, despite us knowing that under-reporting of these offences is a significant problem (Taylor & Gassner, 2010). The same stands true for arson and firesetting literature.

In an attempt to circumvent the problem of poor detection of arson offences, some researchers have widened the sample pool. By choosing to focus on the act of firesetting more broadly, rather than specifically the offence of arson, an increasing number of empirical studies have employed community-based samples. The fact that this was missing from the literature base was identified over a decade ago by Perrin-Wallqvist and Norlander (2003) who suggested there was "a need for studies from normal populations" (p. 152). Recently, three quantitative studies explored the prevalence of firesetting in the general population and the characteristics of those reporting it, in addition to exploring comparisons between a community sample of firesetters and non-firesetters through the use of self-report questionnaires (Gannon & Barrowcliffe, 2012; Barrowcliffe & Gannon, 2015, 2016). Importantly, a self-reported prevalence rate of 11% was found for deliberate (non-convicted) firesetting within the general population (Gannon & Barrowcliffe, 2012), which endorses the important point that not everyone who sets fires is convicted for doing so.

The non-firesetter/firesetter dichotomy

As argued earlier, the categorisation of participants as non-firesetters or firesetters in quantitative research is subjective. In an epidemiological study by Vaughn et al. (2010), one single screening question was used to identify firesetters (as part of a much broader set of psychiatric screening questions), namely: "in your entire life, did you ever start a fire on purpose to destroy someone else's property or just to see it burn?" (p. 3). Such a question is surely open to conjecture and could fail to detect those setting fires for other reasons such as to threaten life or to express oneself.

The screening method employed by Barrowcliffe and Gannon (2016) is much more encompassing. In order to screen their participants as either non-firesetters or firesetters, participants were asked to indicate if they had ever set fires for any of the following reasons: "to annoy other people, to relieve boredom, to create excitement, for insurance purposes, as a result of peer pressure, or to get rid of evidence". Participants were instructed to discount fires set as a child, those which were accidental and those relating to an organised event (p. 387). Even this method of screening could conceivably be flawed. It could lead participants away from considering fires set for other, equally, anti-social purposes, such as to threaten life or to seek revenge. That being said, this approach certainly marks an innovative way forward in addressing the under-representativeness of convicted samples.

In examining researchers' efforts to screen participants into a non-firesetter or firesetter category I am seeking to highlight one fundamental point, namely, that this is extremely difficult. Furthermore, it is subjective to some extent in that the threshold for what one researcher considers to be firesetting could likely differ from the threshold identified by another researcher. In fact, to find an all-encompassing screening method is, in my view, impossible and this is because firesetting (or fire use as I term it) is simply not a categorical phenomenon. Rather, it is dimensional and, thus, any attempt to dichotomise it may not always provide a full picture of how people engage with fire in the real world. The dimensional nature of fire use is the focus of Chapter 4.

Other caveats

There are also other methodological issues with existing quantitative research into arson and firesetting. One such issue relates, broadly, to the draw-backs of using self-report questionnaires in research, which have been widely criticised (Greenwald et al., 2002; Gawronski, LeBel & Peters, 2007). Most notably participants may be inclined to manage the impression that they portray to others by describing themselves in overly positive terms (Paulhus, 1998; p. 1). A handful of pioneering studies have attempted to overcome these issues through employing experimental methods (in the form of computerised tasks) to *implicitly* measure fire-related psychological factors such as fire interest (for examples, see Gallagher-Duffy, MacKay, Duffy, Sullivan-Thomas & Peterson-Badali, 2009; Barrowcliffe, Gannon & Tyler, 2019) – this work is returned to below.

Notwithstanding the aforementioned caveats, the literature base on arson and firesetting is expanding and, particularly in the past few decades, has significantly improved what we know of the behaviour from a psychological perspective. Key findings are reviewed below.

Recidivism and dangerousness

How dangerous are convicted arsonists and others who set fires? Before even starting to answer this question we need to establish what dangerousness means. Interestingly, many authors have tended to equate dangerousness with recidivism, which is dubious practice - returned to below. The question of recidivism (i.e. the rate at which people who have previously set fires go on to set additional fires) is important but it is prudent to note certain limitations of empirical studies, such as the "unsystematic nature of data generation" (Dickens et al., 2009, p. 636). In other words, the methods employed and the way in which recidivism is defined has varied greatly. This has resulted in a vast disparity in reported rates of recidivism, which Brett (2004) found to range from 4 to 60%. For example, rates of 10%, 38% and 60% are cited by Hurley and Monahan (1969), Koson and Dvoskin (1982), and Rice and Harris (1991) respectively, but the operational definition of recidivism varies across studies, with some even including "dangerous smoking" (Geller, Fisher & Bertsch, 1992, p. 147) in their definition. Notwithstanding certain caveats pertaining to the quality of the data, it is prudent to review what we know from recidivism studies because this illuminates the extent of the problem of arson and firesetting.

Some recidivism studies have explored rates for arson/firesetting in comparison to general (i.e. non-arson/firesetting) recidivism. For example, amongst their sample of arsonists, Edwards and Grace (2014) cite a low arson recidivism rate of just over 6%, but a much higher rate for violent and non-violent offending, supporting earlier findings from Rice and Harris (1996). This pattern of higher *general* recidivism, rather than arson-specific recidivism, in samples of convicted arsonists, has been replicated in Australia (Ducat, McEwan & Ogloff, 2015, p. 12). Ostensibly then, this indicates that a convicted arsonist is more likely to recidivate by committing a non-fire related offence than by committing another offence involving fire.

Research into the nature and correlates of recidivism in those who set fires is valuable because it informs clinical practice. For example, it can inform forensic psychologists about the most pertinent factors for consideration in a risk assessment and it can also guide the identification of treatment needs. So far, most of the research into risk factors for arson/firesetting relates to static risk. In other words, the focus has been on aspects of a person's life and presentation which are historical and/or are unlikely to change even with treatment and support. Static risk factors such as a young age at the time of the first firesetting incident, a history of special educational needs or a low Intelligence Quotient (IQ) and a family history of violence and/or substance misuse (Rice & Harris, 1996; Dickens et al., 2009) are thought to be associated with arson/firesetting recidivism.

Further, Edwards and Grace (2014) cite three static variables as being predictive of arson recidivism, namely: being under 18 at the time of the first arson offence, multiple arsons (i.e. multiple counts of arson at the time of the "criterion offence") and prior vandalism offences (p. 224). The optimal predictor in their study was found to be multiple arsons. Of particular pertinence here is the authors' assertion that risk factors for arson are different from those of other offences (p. 226). Similarly, Ducat et al. (2015) identify static variables predictive of arson including multiple arsons at the time of index offence, age at first arson offence and a lifetime history of psychiatric illness. The authors conclude that general anti-sociality, especially from a young age, remains the best predictor of repeat firesetting.

This type of research paves the way for the development of firesetting-specific psychological risk assessment tools. More widely, information gleaned from recidivism research could inform the practice of probation officers, the police and even the FRS through isolating characteristics associated with high recidivism risk, thereby supporting early detection. That being said, when considering risk, static factors (i.e. those which are historical and/or unlikely to change) only tell us part of the story. In my own discipline, best practice dictates that forensic psychologists should also explore what are known as dynamic risk factors, i.e. characteristics of a person which can change, and that these should be the targets for treatment (Douglas & Skeem, 2005) – returned to below.

As referred to earlier, recidivism and dangerousness tend to be treated as synonymous in the forensic psychological literature on firesetting (Dickens et al., 2009). This means that there is a common assumption that those who recidivate more frequently are more dangerous than those who do not. This practice dates back decades, for instance in a 1982 paper Faulk states "when the question of future dangerousness of a patient is discussed, one is asking what is the likelihood of the patient repeating that or a similar offence in a variety of situations" (p. 76). Dickens et al. (2009) challenge this assumption by arguing that recidivism and dangerousness can be mutually exclusive. This is a common-sense viewpoint which can be explained by way of a simple example as follows: imagine two convicted arsonists named Mr. A and Mr. B. Mr. A repeatedly reoffends by setting small fires to litter bins in remote parkland areas where nobody else is around; the fires tend to die down very quickly. In contrast, Mr. B has only one arson re-offence on record which involved setting fire to an inhabited building; all of the residents died in the fire. Who might we consider to be the most dangerous, Mr. A or Mr. B? On the basis of the information available, we could logically surmise that Mr. B; the infrequent recidivator is the more dangerous because of the consequences of his crime. However, Faulk and others would presumably argue that Mr. A is the more dangerous because he has recidivated more often. This example highlights that delineating recidivism and dangerousness is logical and supports the argument for an idiosyncratic approach to the assessment and treatment of people who set fires.

Before moving on to discuss how we think about arson and firesetting behaviour in Chapter 4, a review of the existing literature will continue. Dynamic risk factors, such as psychological characteristics of arsonists and firesetters, according to existing research, are the focus of the next section. To reiterate, existing research tends to refer to people who set fires as firesetters or arsonists and, thus, these are the terms I am referring to within this chapter. It is also important to highlight again that the sub-headings under which this review of the literature is presented are by no means mutually exclusive.

Characteristics of arsonists and firesetters

Characteristics of arsonists and firesetters have attracted the attention of researchers since, at least, the 1950s. Comparisons have been drawn between arsonists/firesetters and people who have committed non-fire-related crimes with a view to isolating similarities and differences. This relates to an ongoing debate which Gannon et al. (2013) refer to as the *generalist and specialist hypothesis* (p. 4). Proponents of the generalist viewpoint see those who set fires as sharing much in common with those who have committed other forms of crime, whereas supporters of the specialist school of thought assert that those who set fires present a different picture to their violent, non-violent and sexually violent counterparts. For forensic practitioners, such as forensic psychologists, there is great value in exploring this debate. If people who are in prison for setting fires are very similar, psychologically, to other sub-groups in prison then surely a generic assessment and treatment strategy is sufficient. However, if they are psychologically different in some way, this makes the case for a better-tailored approach.

The existing firesetting literature offers no definitive conclusion to the aforementioned debate because research has found both similarities and differences when arsonists/firesetters are compared to counterparts with other offending backgrounds. Even in the 1990s, however, some support for the specialist hypothesis had already begun to emerge. For instance, Rice and Harris (1996) state "firesetting is quite distinct from both violent and other non-violent crime", adding that it is most different from violent offending (p. 373). The fact that even *some* differences have been found surely supports the specialist side of the argument and, thus, makes the case for a specialist approach to the assessment and treatment of people who set fires. Let us now turn to a review of the mixed findings.

Some authors claim that low assertiveness might distinguish firesetters from people who commit other crimes (Jackson et al., 1987) whereas others have found no difference (Day, 2001; Gannon et al., 2013). Similarly, self-reported self-esteem has been explored, with some studies finding that firesetters score lower than people who have committed other crimes (Duggan & Shine, 2001; Gannon et al., 2013) but others cite no difference (Day, 2001). Other psychological characteristics have received varying degrees of research attention in the firesetting literature, including impulsivity (Ritchie & Huff, 1999; Dolan, Millington & Park, 2002; Labree, Nijman, Van Marle & Rassin, 2010), anger related cognition (Gannon et al., 2013), emotional regulation (Gannon et al., 2013), increased hostility (Hagenauw, Karsten, Akkerman-Bouwsema, de Jager, & Lancel, 2015), and poor social and relational skills (Hagenauw et al., 2015).

Compellingly, recent research has explored *fire-specific* constructs in firesetters. Identification with fire, interest in serious and everyday fires, attitudes condoning firesetting as normal and fire safety awareness have been explored and four of the five have been found to distinguish between firesetters and non-firesetters (Gannon et al., 2013; Ó Ciardha et al., 2015). Of particular potential is the study of fire interest (Barrowcliffe et al., 2019), namely, a specific interest in fire as characterised by an inclination to attend to fire (or fire-related stimuli). Research into constructs such as this can inform the work of practitioners seeking to identify characteristics which might raise a service user's risk and, thus, which require targeted treatment.

Thus far, the vast majority of research into fire-specific constructs, such as fire interest, has employed self-report questionnaires. Self-report instruments are *explicit* measures in that they ask participants, directly, about their views, beliefs or attitudes on a particular topic. The preference for questionnaire-based designs is understandable given the large sample sizes it can yield and the pressure on psychological researchers to produce research with high statistical power (Sassenberg & Ditrich, 2019). However, there are drawbacks to this form of data collection as referred to earlier. In response to this, *implicit* measures of fire-specific constructs, such as fire interest, have been employed recently. This method is advantageous because it does not demand introspection on the part of a participant (Gawronski et al., 2007, p. 181).

One example of an implicit measure is the emotional Stroop task, employed by Gallagher-Duffy et al. (2009). This study measured information-processing bias for pictorial fire-related stimuli in a sample of 98 male adolescents, including those with firesetting needs and two control groups. Findings indicate that the firesetters were more distracted by fire-related stimuli, and thus, more interested in it. Barrowcliffe et al. (2019) used a different implicit measure – a fire-specific Lexical Decision Task (LDT) – to explore fire-related cognition in a sample of 84 adults. Overall, comparisons in reaction times between self-reported firesetter participants and non-firesetters were as expected, suggesting the relevance of certain cognitions in firesetting. Curiously, however, firesetters' reaction times on the fire interest LDT were *slower* than those for non-firesetters, which was contrary to the hypothesis; this requires further investigation.

Whilst the research discussed above typically involves comparisons between firesetters and non-firesetters, other studies have sought to compare different sub-types of firesetter. One approach has been to compare similarities and differences between "pure arsonists [and] non-pure arsonists" (Lindberg et al., 2005; p. 5), i.e. those who have *only* committed arson and those with a more versatile criminal history. Amongst other differences, Lindberg et al. (2005) found that pure arsonists are more likely to have a diagnosis of psychotic disorder and to have cognitive difficulties, whereas personality disorder diagnoses are more common in non-pure arsonists. In a similar study based in Australia, Ducat et al. (2013) found that exclusive firesetters are more commonly women and are older at the time of the first conviction when compared to two other sub-groups, namely those who are predominantly firesetters and those with a mixture of offence-types on record (p. 552).

In my view, research exploring sub-types of people who set fires should have as much influence on practice as that which draws comparisons between those who light fires and other convicted groups. If the specialist hypothesis is to be accepted, then generic approaches to assessment and treatment are not appropriate for those who set fires. However, if we also accept that people who light fires are themselves a heterogeneous group (Thompson et al., 2015), then it might be necessary to tailor our approach even more precisely to cater for different sub-types. For instance, it may be the case that people who have only lit one fire require different treatment to recidivists and that those *only* committing arson have different psychological needs to those of people who have a versatile offending history. Indeed, the heterogeneity of firesetters is outlined through five trajectories in the M-TTAF (Gannon et al., 2012) – see below.

Despite the shortcomings and limitations discussed above, research into the demographic, criminal and psychological characteristics of firesetters has been integral in informing the practice of forensic psychologists and other forensic practitioners. Furthermore, empirical work paves the way for the development and refinement of theoretical perspectives, which are important for guiding assessment and treatment. The most influential are discussed below.

Theoretical perspectives

In the previous section, empirical research was reviewed. In the following section work which has specifically sought to classify arsonists and/or firesetters is outlined. As with the empirical literature, theoretical work uses the terms arsonist or firesetter and, thus, these terms are used below when citing this existing literature. The structure of the following section is broadly chronological to reflect how theoretical understanding has evolved over time.

From typologies to multi-factor theories

One of the first attempts to classify those who set fires are known as typologies (Gannon & Pina, 2010). These classificatory systems adopt either an *inductive* or *deductive* approach, the former being the most popular (Dickens & Sugarman, 2012). A key premise of inductive typologies is that firesetters can be categorised into subtypes on the basis of the motivation underpinning their crime, in addition to other characteristics (Dickens & Sugarman, 2012; p. 50). There are a number of issues with early inductive typologies, not least the dubiousness of isolating one specific motivation for a crime.

Furthermore, Dickens and Sugarman (2012) highlight "there is little evidence that the development of category headings for classificatory purposes has involved any more than *thinking about* the data" (p. 50). The problems with typologies led to the emergence of multi-factor theoretical perspectives on arson and firesetting.

Until recently there were only two multifactor theories (Fritzon, 2012, p. 29). The first of these, the functional analysis model (Jackson et al., 1987) explains recidivistic arson as a function of certain antecedents, followed by behaviourally reinforcing consequences. The model has clinical utility; however, it has little empirical support (Gannon & Pina, 2010). The dynamic behaviour model (Fineman, 1995) shares commonalities with the work of Jackson et al. It, too, addresses historical factors which could contribute to arson, the role of reinforcement and also the environment but Fineman's perspective also advances on the work of Jackson et al, for example, by referring to the role of cognition (Fritzon, 2012).

The two aforementioned theories were the first to approach firesetting from a multi-factor perspective. In my own practice as a forensic psychologist, I use them to make sense of a firesetting offence, not only when conducting assessments but also in working therapeutically with those who set fires. However, they are limited in scope and do not provide adequate coverage of all potentially relevant risk factors (Gannon et al., 2013). There was, therefore, a need for a more comprehensive theory, and thus, the multi-trajectory theory of adult firesetting (M-TTAF; Gannon et al., 2012) was proposed.

The M-TTAF, it is argued by its proponents, builds on the strengths of the aforementioned theories by Jackson et al. (1987) and Fineman (1995) and is structured as a two-tiered theoretical framework. Tier one relates to the aetiology of firesetting, including multiple interconnected factors such as biological predisposition, culture, context, the role of social learning and psychological characteristics. The M-TTAF expands on factors such as fire-specific cognition, which is one of many advances upon its predecessors. Another key addition is the explanation of the maintenance and desistance of firesetting (Gannon et al., 2012). Tier two of the M-TTAF comprises five prototypical trajectories, based on patterns of characteristics leading to firesetting (Gannon et al., 2012). In brief, these are: (i) *anti-social cognition* – individuals who set fires within the context of a generally anti-social lifestyle; (ii) *grievance* – those who light fires as a form of revenge, and for whom characteristics such as hostility are of relevance; (iii) *fire interest* – those for whom fire acts as a coping mechanism by increasing or decreasing physiological arousal; (iv) *emotionally expressive/need for recognition* – individuals whose primary risk factors involve communication-skill deficits; and (v) *multi-faceted* – those who have a generally anti-social lifestyle but who also have a particular interest in fire.

Owing to its contemporary status the M-TTAF is yet to be fully evaluated. A recent study into the characteristics of firesetters admitted for a pre-trial psychiatric assessment in the Netherlands offers partial support (Dalhuisen, Koenraadt & Liem, 2017. However, the clusters of characteristics discovered by Dalhuisen et al., do not map on to the M-TTAF trajectories exactly; this raises the need for further work into the M-TTAF specifically, but it could also hint at cultural differences in firesetting.

From a practice perspective, the M-TTAF guides understanding of a firesetter's presentation. It can be used flexibly and supports an idiosyncratic approach. As mentioned above, one of its strengths is the attention paid to the role of cognition in firesetting. The central role of cognition, for instance in the form of *implicit theories* (ITs)[1] has been evidenced in relation to other crimes such as rape (for example, Polaschek & Gannon, 2004). However, until recently, it had not been addressed in firesetters. Empirical research has now begun to explore cognition in firesetters, including relevant ITs (Ó Ciardha & Gannon, 2012) and cognitive scripts (Butler & Gannon, 2015, 2020).

Whilst the M-TTAF offers a broad framework for understanding firesetting, other theoretical work has focused specifically on a firesetting offence.

Offence chain theories

Offence chains in this case are micro-level theories of adult firesetting, designed to explain the offence, specifically, including those perpetrated by mentally disordered (Tyler, Gannon, Lockerbie, King, Dickens & De Burca, 2014) and non-mentally disordered (Barnoux, Gannon & Ó Ciardha, 2015) firesetters. The theories are based on data from qualitative studies involving interviews with firesetters either residing in prison or in secure psychiatric units. Tyler et al., and Barnoux et al., identify a four-phase offence chain process comprising: (i) background factors; (ii) adulthood; (iii) the pre-offence phase; and (iv) offence and post-offence phase.

Given that much of the existing quantitative work cited previously focusses on firesetting as a single construct, the deconstruction of this behaviour into stages offers a more nuanced insight. A particular strength of both offence chain theories is the consideration of the post-offence stage which has received very little attention in the existing psychological literature but which might be particularly illuminating with respect to the motivation for a firesetting incident and the psychological presentation of those who set fires. For example, whether or not a perpetrator remains at the scene of a fire or, indeed, returns to the scene at a later date, might be highly informative for clinicians seeking to assess and reduce risk. Tyler et al. (2014) and Barnoux et al. (2015) also discuss different pathways into a firesetting offence, which again is of help to forensic practitioners.

A focus on risk

One commonality which all of the above empirical and theoretical contributions share is their focus on risk, risk factors and pathological behaviour. A focus on such topics has, historically, been typical of research and practice in forensic psychology (Rogers, 2000). Over the past few decades, however, a strong argument has emerged for a more balanced appraisal of forensic service users and, indeed, the behaviour in which they engage. More specifically, there has been a call for protective factors to be addressed (for discussions see Towl & Crighton, 1996; Ward, 2017). Protective factors are those characteristics which mitigate a person's risk of committing a crime, or to which desistance has been attributed. In other words, in addition to identifying what is 'wrong' with a service user and their behaviour in an attempt to remove it, we should be striving to identify and build on the individual's strengths (Horsley, 2020). Encouragingly, consideration of protective factors is an increasing feature of research and practice in the forensic arena in general (for examples, see Heffernan & Ward, 2017; de Vries Robbé, de Vogel, Koster & Bogaerts, 2015; Ullrich & Coid, 2011). However, there is a need to address it more pointedly in relation to people who set fires. The utility of a strengths-based approach in understanding arson and firesetting is returned to throughout this book because it underpins the reconceptualisation which I am calling for.

Implications

The existing firesetting literature reflects progress, albeit slow, from both an empirical and theoretical perspective. Research has improved our understanding of the risk and dangerousness of people who light fires, as well as demographic and psychological characteristics, which has genuine clinical utility. Research drawing comparisons between sub-types of people who set fires also shows potential. For instance, people who have set only one fire might differ from those with a string of fire-related incidents on record and, thus, we should adopt an idiosyncratic approach.

Crucially, it is now widely acknowledged that people who set fires are a heterogeneous group, whose needs may vary greatly. This is important from an assessment and treatment perspective. More specifically, given that there are no validated risk assessment tools for use with those who light fires (Watt &

Ong, 2016) nor any accredited treatment programmes (Palmer et al., 2007; Bell, 2016; Tyler et al., 2018), research supporting an idiosyncratic approach to clinical work is very important. It is noteworthy that, so far, I have focused mainly on how the existing literature can inform practitioners' work with service users in the CJS. In later chapters, the discussion will be broadened to consider early interventions.

Summary

Even though I am arguing that studying the *misuse* of fire does not tell the whole story about the human-fire relationship it is, nevertheless, still one important *part* of the story. Despite the progress that has been made, limitations with the literature remain, including a failure by some to define terms, such as firesetting clearly enough. Furthermore, we know very little about women who set fires (for reviews see Gannon, 2010; Gannon et al., 2012; Fritzon & Miller, 2016) and empirical findings are largely based on specialist samples which is dubious owing to low arson detection rates (Daykin & Hamilton, 2012). The slow emergence of community-based research is, therefore, encouraging (for example, Gannon & Barrowcliffe, 2012; Barrowcliffe & Gannon, 2015, 2016). Fundamentally, much of the research being published currently is of a similar nature. The literature is dominated by quantitative research seeking to categorise participants as non-firesetters or firesetters. In addition, the published literature tends to be uni-disciplinary, which I argue leads to an over-simplification of fire-related behaviour. Perhaps the root of some of the aforementioned issues is much more fundamental than specific methodological flaws. It seems that the over-focus on risk is problematic but even more broadly, perhaps the way we think about criminal behaviour in general and firesetting specifically is the crux of the problem.

Note

1 **Implicit Theory:** People's understanding of their own "beliefs, desires, needs and behaviors" (Polaschek & Gannon, 2004, p. 300).

Understanding fire use   4

Overview

In Chapter 2, our species' long and complex history with fire was discussed, including fire's use as a tool for survival, its symbolic importance and its entertaining qualities. I term adaptive use of fire *non-criminalised fire use* - defined as fire-related behaviour, which is considered to adhere to laws, rules and social norms, is generally seen as justifiable and is not underpinned by malicious or reckless intent. In the previous chapter, existing psychological literature on the misuse of fire in the form of arson and firesetting was reviewed. I term this *criminalised fire use* – defined as fire-related behaviour, which is considered to violate laws, rules and social norms, is generally considered to be non-justifiable, and which is likely to have been enacted with malicious or reckless intent.

What, specifically, constitutes non-criminalised and criminalised fire use? I suggest that seeking to delineate the two is not particularly helpful because of the subjectivity involved. This also applies to the previously discussed non-firesetter/ firesetter dichotomy. Below, an alternative conceptualisation is presented. First, however, this chapter will explore dichotomies more generally, in reference to human behaviour.

A meaningful dichotomy?

In the UK, the decision about what is 'acceptable' and 'unacceptable' behaviour is ultimately determined by the legal system. Arson is a legal term, which relates to the specific criminal act of intentionally or recklessly setting fire to property

DOI: 10.4324/9780367808648-4

or woodland area (Dickens et al., 2009, p. 3). It is defined by the Criminal Damage Act 1971, of which section 1 (3) stipulates that any criminal damage caused by fire should be classed, and charged, as arson (Averill, 2010). Since 2008 the offence has been subdivided into three: (i) simple arson, (ii) arson reckless as to whether life was endangered, and; (iii) arson with intent to endanger life. Within this classification the level of severity differs, with simple arson being the least serious and arson with intent the most severe.

Legal systems tend to use categorical assumptions, such as 'not guilty' or 'guilty' but the world is surely much more nuanced than that. This is why the terms I am proposing (i.e. non-criminalised and criminalised) seek to reflect social rules and norms, as well as legislation. Heyman (2013) notes the "complicated and ambiguous terrain between legality and illegality" (p. 322). Likewise, Botoeva (2019) refers to "the grey area between legal and illegal practices" and adds that "it is not always possible to separate the legal from the illegal and therefore clearly demarcate the boundaries between them". Botoeva concludes that "the notion of what is legal and illegal, stated and formalised by states, can be contested by other actors" (p. 68); a point with which I agree entirely. In other words, what a state or country defines as illegal may not always be the same as how that behaviour is viewed by the general public. Botoeva writes about the role of language in legitimising the practice of hashish production in the mountainous regions of north-east Kyrgyzstan. According to Botoeva changes in the language used to refer to this behaviour means that to some people in the population, the harvesting of hashish is considered socially acceptable despite the fact that the state considers it illegal (p. 68).

Consideration of how the legal system defines a particular behaviour in contrast to how it is defined from a social science perspective is important. Before moving on to expand on my conceptualisation of fire use, it is prudent to broaden the discussion about defining behaviour from fire use to anti-social/ criminal acts more generally. Doing so elucidates why it is so challenging to reach consensus about what is deemed to be acceptable and unacceptable behaviour in the social sciences.

The judgements we make about the acceptability of a person's behaviour are likely influenced by a myriad of factors including culture, societal norms and moral stance (Botoeva, 2019). In the criminological literature, Andrews and Bonta (2014) epitomise this point perfectly by highlighting the many alternative, and arguably conflicting, approaches to defining criminal behaviour. Andrews and Bonta list the following definitions: (i) *legal* – acts failing to abide by state law; (ii) *moral* – the breaching of religious and moral norms; (iii) *social* – the breaching of social norms and; (iv) *psychological* – behaviour which causes pain or loss for others. Nutt, King, Saulsbury and Blakemore (2007) echo a similar sentiment in their approach to scrutinising the classification of drugs in the UK.

They assert that the existing legal classification (i.e. class A, B and C) is insufficient because it fails to account for the nuanced considerations in relation to the effects of drugs. As an alternative, Nutt et al. (2007) suggest that drugs should be classified on the basis of how much harm they cause, through consideration of three factors: (i) physical harm caused to the drug user; (ii) the tendency of the drug to induce dependence; and (iii) the effect of the drug on families, communities and society. The culmination of the work of Nutt et al. (2007) is a nine-category matrix through which a drug can be rated with respect to its level of harm. This elucidates the point that human behaviour is much more complex than a simple legal/illegal dichotomy, at least to those looking at it from a social science viewpoint. Indeed, there is a whole literature base in cultural criminology which considers the concept of deviant leisure activities (for example, see Smith & Raymen, 2018). Whilst such activities may not be illegal per se, they can still lead to a variety of different forms of harm (Smith & Raymen, 2018; p. 65), and this points to the value of a dimensional perspective.

What the work outlined above highlights is the many grey areas in deciding what is acceptable and unacceptable. Lawyers might argue that legality supersedes anything else but is this always a cut-and-dried case? Consider, for example, the moral and religious importance that people of particular cultures and faiths living in the UK place on not eating certain meats, despite the fact that meat-eating is not against the law in the UK. Another particularly contemporary example relates to the way in which people's behaviour was viewed during the COVID-19 worldwide pandemic, which begun in the year 2020. During periods which came to be known as 'lockdown' in the UK, the British Government urged members of the public not only to abide by the rules, which were written in the law (such as not socialising with large groups of people indoors), but also to behave in the 'spirit' of the rules (such as 'staying local' for one's daily exercise). The problem here is that how to abide by the spirit of the rules is a highly subjective matter. There are manifold other examples of the conflict between what constitutes right or wrong and such a conflict applies just as well to fire use – returned to below.

As Andrews and Bonta's list demonstrates, how a behaviour is appraised can be dependent on many factors beyond what is captured in the written law. However, even the written law is not without subjectivity. Schur (1969), for example, makes reference to the variability of the law from country to country. For that reason, he argues, the law cannot possibly be the sole determinant of what is criminal (or non-criminal for that matter). This supports the argument that behaviour is socially constructed and that it can be difficult to define because of the many grey areas. This is exemplified in a sociological concept termed the *carnival of crime* (Presdee, 2000), through which Presdee discusses the unclear boundary between carnival and crime and how one can morph into the other.

To summarise so far, it is difficult to delineate what is acceptable or unacceptable/criminal or non-criminal/illegal or legal behaviour. Even where we believe the law is clear-cut, laws vary greatly from country to country and legality is only one of many considerations for social scientists trying to make sense of behaviour. So what of fire use specifically? Is it possible to neatly categorise it as non-criminalised and criminalised (or non-firesetting and firesetting for that matter)? I argue not.

Non-criminalised and criminalised fire use

In Chapter 3, the practice of execution by burning in England was referred to. I posited that public perception about the acceptability of this has likely changed over time. Presdee (2005) highlights another example of a change in public perceptions – the lighting of bonfires for 5th November celebrations in the UK. He notes that in the past this practice was viewed as dangerous, whereas now they are commercialised events, which are properly regulated. Presdee emphasises here that the passage of time, along with culture, social norms and moral stance, can determine the judgements one makes about the permissibility of another's behaviour. But what of other forms of fire use?

Consider a neighbour who decides to use an outdoor chiminea to entertain friends in their garden. Whilst generally not against the law it could be criminalised by those in adjacent homes. In other words, it might be viewed as a breach of social norms or etiquette because of the inconvenience of the smoke it produces and, indeed, the potential for the fire to get out of control. On a much larger scale is the example of burning fossil fuels. This might, by some, be categorised as criminalised because of its destabilising impact on the Earth's atmospheric conditions (Pyne, 2019). What these examples show is that whether certain forms of fire use are socially constructed as non-criminalised or criminalised might vary from person to person and, indeed, culture to culture. An unpublished MSc thesis which I supervised adds some preliminary support to this argument. Hope (2018) interviewed 16 participants about the attributes they consider as important when distinguishing between two forms of fire use – legitimate or illegitimate (broadly speaking these terms correspond to non-criminalised and criminalised respectively, which I have since come to use as an alternative). Crucially, Hope found no definitive binary framework through which to categorise fire use as one or the other.

To complicate matters further, not only is it difficult to categorise fire use as non-criminalised or criminalised but there are many gradations of each. We only need to return to an earlier example to see the logic behind this argument, namely setting fire to a litter bin in a deserted public park and setting fire to an inhabited dwelling. Both of these acts could conceivably be considered criminalised, however, the latter is surely *more* criminalised than the former. Therefore, even where two acts are obviously criminalised (or, indeed, non-criminalised), there are different degrees.

I argue that it is not possible to neatly categorise fire use because the behaviour is simply more nuanced than that. Fire use can vary on two levels. The first of these relates to variability across a population. Indeed, fire use might differ between different communities, cultures, religions, nations, whole continents and so on. The second level relates to variability across a single person's lifespan and might range from entirely appropriate (non-criminalised) to acquiring an arson conviction (criminalised). Both of these levels of variability are perfectly epitomised by participants in my research (Horsley, 2020; discussed in detail in Chapter 5). Across a sample of 24 UK-based adults, forms of fire use varied vastly from the lighting of candles, to ritualistic and religious uses through to arson convictions. Similarly, each individual participant's fire use typically varied across their lifespan. For example, Viv who is currently serving a prison sentence for arson says this of her offence which involved setting fire to the victim's flat: "I just started throwing clothes in and then I watched it burn for a few minutes". In contrast, however, she also recalled a seemingly non-criminalised form of fire use earlier in her life: "when you're just sitting on the sofa and the fireplace is burning; it's quite a pretty scene". The diversity in individuals' fire use is highly significant. It suggests that in our work with those who have firesetting convictions it is prudent to consider healthy interactions with fire as well as their offence/s. This is because *all* interactions with fire might contribute to the relationship they have formed with it.

The discussion earlier about the difficulty in delineating legally and socially acceptable and non-acceptable behaviour, along with the variation in fire use (i.e. across a whole population and a single person's lifespan) has led me to propose that it should be viewed as sitting on a continuum – the Continuum of Fire Use (CoFU; Horsley, 2020, 2021).

The Continuum of Fire Use (CoFU)

Rather than relying on dichotomies such as non-firesetting/firesetting, acceptable/non-acceptable or legal/illegal and so on, we should consider fire use as sitting on a continuum – the CoFU (see Figure 4.1). This reconceptualisation was the premise of my doctoral research conducted between 2014 and 2019. Subsequently, Tyler and Gannon (2020) have also noted the need for a dimensional understanding of fire use, which demonstrates that this idea is gaining traction.

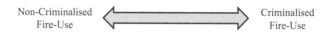

Figure 4.1 The Continuum of Fire Use (CoFU).

The CoFU has two poles. At one pole sits non-criminalised fire use and at the opposing end of the continuum is criminalised fire use, which includes firesetting and arson crimes. The CoFU can be applied to the conceptualisation of fire use on the two levels outlined above, i.e. to represent the variation across a whole population *and* across a single person's lifespan. Crucially, the position of different forms of fire use along the continuum is a subjective judgement, which itself serves to reinforce the very essence of the dimensional argument.

The CoFU elucidates the *fluidity* of human fire use and signifies that one person's lifetime use can vacillate along the continuum. It is the broad conceptualisation on which I have based a *theory* of fire use – outlined in Chapter 5. As outlined in Chapter 3, the psychological literature, thus far, has focussed solely on arson and firesetting and so has clustered around the criminalised pole of the continuum. This means that our knowledge of fire use as a holistic construct is limited. Seeking to understand the CoFU in its entirety offers a novel and practical way forward.

The dimensionality idea already features in other areas of psychology, of course. For example, a dimensional understanding of personality disorder is favoured above a categorical approach (Livesley, 2007). More specifically, it is important to note that the idea that fire has 'two sides', i.e. positives and negatives, is not entirely new either. For example, in her work with young people who set fires, Foster (2020b) refers to "good fires and bad fires" and recommends the use of a fire safety book written by Mary Flahavin on the topic (p. 66). Likewise, the continuum, when applied to fire, is not a wholly new concept. Flynn (2009; as cited in Britt, 2011) developed a continuum of youth fire-related behaviour model which is a speculative depiction of how risk in juvenile fire use can increase from fire play and curiosity to delinquent and pathological behaviour. Flynn's work, however, is designed purely for juveniles and is related specifically to risk. The CoFU, contrastingly, is intended to apply to fire use more broadly.

The CoFU is intended to be both a conceptual framework, i.e. a way of thinking about fire use and also a practical tool for clinicians working with those who set fires in the criminal justice and health care systems. Its premise is that we can learn more about the most extreme and maladaptive fire-related behaviour (deliberate firesetting/arson) by looking at the many gradations of fire use, including adaptive forms. This is a deceptively simple concept, which is analogous to other areas of forensic psychology, such as clinical practice with those who have a record of sexual offending. In examining risk in a person convicted of a sexual offence using a tool called the Risk of Sexual Violence Protocol (RSVP; Hart et al., 2003), one of the characteristics a clinician must assess is sexual deviance, which is defined as "a stable pattern of deviant sexual arousal" (p. 62). According to the RSVP administration manual, the clinician must consider the degree to which deviant interest is present in the examinee's case, and, crucially this should be appraised "relative to non-deviant sexual interests" (p. 62). In other words, the clinician should consider *non*-deviance as a baseline so that they can make a judgement about the extent to which sexual *deviance* is relevant in that particular case. This is not always straightforward, of course because, in reality, like fire use, sexual interest is a dimensional construct. Nevertheless, exactly the same principle can be applied to fire use, namely, in order to fully understand deviant use of fire, i.e. fire-setting/arson, we must have an understanding of the array of behaviours which constitute non-deviant use, i.e. non-criminalised fire use.

Understanding the spectrum of fire use has clinical utility, expounded upon within subsequent chapters. In brief, first, clinicians should consider adaptive forms of fire use, alongside maladaptive forms, occurring throughout the life of a person who sets fires. Secondly, the psychological factors associated with *healthy* fire use could be a core target of rehabilitative treatment. Thirdly, and of most importance, what we learn about healthy fire use and, more broadly, healthy relationships with fire should be the blueprint for early interventions with young people.

The notion of considering healthy and positive aspects (i.e. non-criminalised) of fire use is broadly consistent with the move in forensic psychology practice from a sole focus on risk to one which also considers positive characteristics, i.e. protective factors (for discussions see Towl & Crighton, 1996; Ward, 2017). This shift in focus is underpinned by principles of *positive psychology* (for reviews see Seligman & Csikszentmihalyi, 2000; Seligman, Steen, Park & Peterson, 2005). Its premise is that we should focus our attention on an individual's strengths and positive characteristics, such as the "capacity for love and vocation… interpersonal skill… perseverance, altruism… and work ethic" (Seligman & Csikszentmihalyi, 2000, p. 5). Positive psychology has been heavily promoted in the forensic academic literature (for example, see Heffernan & Ward, 2017; Ward, 2017). It is also the basis of a well-established model which promotes desistance in those who previously committed crime – the Good Lives Model (GLM; see Ward & Brown, 2004 for an overview). The GLM proposes that all humans are motivated to meet a set of "primary human goods" (Ward & Brown, 2004, p. 246), which for our purpose, could be loosely thought of as intrinsic life goals. According to the GLM, those who commit crime have a tendency to pursue their goals maladaptively. The model, and the rehabilitative interventions predicated upon it, promote supporting those who have committed a crime to pursue goals in a more adaptive and pro-social manner.

My argument about taking a more holistic view of fire use aligns with the positive psychology ethos. I am suggesting that fire use is a dimensional construct and, as such, we should seek to understand the whole dimension rather than solely negative aspects of the human–fire relationship. In the spirit of a holistic approach, we must surely appreciate the longevity of this relationship and how it has evolved over time because this forms the basis of how we view and interact with fire today. Psychology cannot possibly address these matters as a standalone discipline which is why I am calling for an interdisciplinary approach.

Summary

Although UK law generally considers behaviour as 'legal' or 'illegal', social scientists study it at a much more nuanced level and so examining the different granularities of behaviour ranging from what we might consider appropriate to inappropriate is a more fruitful method. This thinking relates to a whole host of different actions but it was applied, specifically, to fire use above. In this chapter, the CoFU has been presented as a new conceptualisation of fire use. The CoFU underpins a theory predicated on my own research (Horsley, 2020), which is outlined in the following chapter.

A preliminary theory of fire use

5

Overview

Predicated on the Continuum of Fire Use (CoFU) framework, the Continuum of Fire Use Theory (CoFUT) was developed through my doctoral research spanning 2014 to 2019 (see Horsley, 2020). In presenting this as a theory, I should highlight that there are different types of theory in psychology. Ward, Polaschek and Beech (2006) discuss three *levels*, which essentially relate to their degree of granularity. Level one is the most all-encompassing type of theory, otherwise termed multi-faceted. Level two is described as a single-factor theory and level three is a theory which relates to one specific behaviour, such as a single instance of fire use or one arson offence. The CoFUT is arguably best thought of as a level two theory in that, predominantly, it explores *psychological* aspects of fire use. Naturally, psychology is the main focus given my background and experience; however, the theory is informed by multi-disciplinary viewpoints (such as those reflected in previous chapters). It is important to emphasise that the CoFUT is a preliminary theory. It is based on one, albeit in-depth, qualitative study and so more data are required to refine it. The research through which the CoFUT was developed is outlined below, starting with my methodological approach.

Methodology

There is a dearth of qualitative research in psychology within the arson and fire-setting literature. Furthermore, as previously highlighted, until now, research has

DOI: 10.4324/9780367808648-5

focused on firesetting rather than fire *use* as a broader, dimensional, construct. These gaps provided the rationale for my doctoral research, which included a data-driven qualitative study of fire use. An abbreviated version of Grounded Theory (GT; Willig, 2013) and more specifically a constructivist approach to GT (Charmaz, 1990) informed data collection and analysis. More detail on the approach and method can be found in Horsley (2020).

I employed purposive sampling (for explanations, see Robinson, 2014; Etikan, Musa & Alkassim, 2016) to identify people with relevant experience of fire for my study. Participants were recruited through a combination of word of mouth (which is known as 'snowball sampling' – referred to by Hood, 2007) and making direct contact (via email) with groups whom I considered relevant, for example, fire performing groups, as well as through approaching prisons in my local area. I aimed to capture a sample of participants with fire-related experiences spanning the whole CoFU, including those sitting at both poles; this is why I not only approached people residing in the community but also those serving prison sentences for arson / with institutional firesetting on record.

I arrived at a sample of 24 adults (nine identifying as men and 15 as women) who were interviewed about their experiences of fire use. For the purpose of this study, 12 participants were identified as predominantly criminalised fire users and 12 predominantly non-criminalised, in accordance with their primary (i.e. most frequent) use/s of fire across the lifespan. Criminalised participants were residing in prison at the time of interview and had firesetting offences and/or institutional firesetting on record. Non-criminalised participants were based in the community and had no firesetting offences or cautions on record. It is important to note that, consistent with the continuum conceptualisation, it was not my intention to form two separate participant categories. Rather, I sought to secure a diverse sample with respect to fire use experiences. Broadly speaking, each participant could be seen as clustering around one of the two poles of the CoFU on the basis of their primary use/s of fire. Therefore, when commentating on the data (below) I will refer to 'forms' of non-criminalised and criminalised fire use because, for brevity, we can consider most types of fire use to be closer to one pole of the continuum than the other. However, in reality, there was vast variability in each of my participants' experiences. Alongside their primary use of fire, each participant reported a range of fire-related experiences. This supports the dimensional way of thinking. My participants' fire use experiences include:

- Functional use – cooking food over fire, the use of fire to keep warm or to complete a task, such as welding;
- Recreational use – this broad category comprises the lighting of bonfires, campfires, candles, fireworks, coal fires and log burners all for the primary purpose of enjoyment;

- Vocational use – the use of fire by artists who are paid to entertain with fire, such as fire jugglers and fire breathers;
- Spiritual and ritualistic use – rituals and ceremonies, for example, the use of fire to cleanse / ward off evil;
- Religious use – the lighting of candles and fires, as well as the burning of objects for religious purposes;
- Self-harm through the use of fire (i.e. by burning one's skin);
- Reckless fire play, including attempts to run through bonfires, aiming fireworks at people and burning objects over a fire (such as childhood toys);
- Setting fire to outdoor public spaces, namely parks / grassland;
- Setting fire to vehicles;
- Setting fire to residential buildings (including houses and flats).

Interviews with each of my 24 participants were audio-recorded, transcribed and analysed (see Horsley, 2020 for details); the findings are discussed below.

Findings: the Continuum of Fire Use Theory (CoFUT)

Three core themes were identified, which relate to the psychology of participants' lifelong fire use, which I refer to as participants' relationship with fire. These themes form the basis of the CoFUT, which is presented in Figure 5.1. I have chosen to present the CoFUT diagrammatically, alongside the narrative description of themes below, for a number of reasons. Firstly, through my experience as both a lecturer and a practitioner I have come to recognise the importance of making information accessible. Some of us are visual learners, whereas others might prefer to deal with written information (Dobson, 2009). Not only is this relevant for students and scholars but also for clinicians who might choose to draw upon the CoFUT in their work with forensic service users. In my practice I have regularly incorporated pictures and diagrams to aid understanding and, as such, I suggest that Figure 5.1 could be helpful in supporting people who set fires to develop insight into their lifelong relationship with fire. The latter point is key here, namely, that the CoFUT represents the psychology of the human-fire relationship as a whole, rather than solely a firesetting offence. Secondly, the diagrammatic representation enables me to highlight interconnections and mechanisms between the core themes in the CoFUT, for example the process of reinforcement, which is depicted by the two-way arrows and the fluid nature of fire use (both *between* different people and, indeed, *across* one person's life span), which is denoted by the continuums along the bottom and top of the diagram.

In the remainder of this chapter, the CoFUT is discussed, along with the data on which it is based. It is important to protect the anonymity of my participants

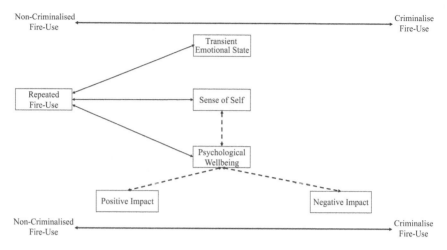

Figure 5.1 Diagrammatic representation of the CoFUT.

who willingly gave their time to share stories and so pseudonyms are used in every case and no identifiable information is included. As I present the CoFUT, I will also indicate support for each of its themes from the existing inter-disciplinary literature.

The CoFUT consists of three core themes: (i) *Transitory Emotional State*, (ii) *Sense of Self*, and (iii) *Psychological Wellbeing*, each of which is discussed below, along with their respective sub-themes. As referred to above, the CoFUT captures psychological factors underpinning the human-fire relationship. These three factors (themes) along with how they interconnect are reviewed below.

Transitory Emotional State

This CoFUT theme relates to the immediate and short-term emotional benefits of engaging with fire use from my participants' perspective. The transitory nature of these benefits characterises this theme in that changes are relatively fleeting and only last as long as a particular instance of fire use or for not long afterwards. The theme is separated into two sub-themes: *Immediate Gratification* and *Mediator*, each of which is expounded below.

Immediate Gratification

This sub-theme is so-called because it describes the way in which fire use *directly* and *immediately* affects participants' physiological state in a positive way.

Participants speak of fire's stimulating properties, for example, by increasing their level of arousal in the form of an "adrenaline rush" according to Connor or a quickening of the heart rate as Clarissa says here: "my heart just races and my stomach's full on giddy". Indeed, Kimmy uses fire medicinally and says she deliberately engages with fire when she needs an energy boost: "maybe I just need a little bit of a boost of something, I'll often put a candle on because it's that spark that seems to ignite the energy again". Some participants make reference to becoming aroused through risky interactions with fire, for example, Rory says: "you put an aerosol can on a fire; it goes bang. It makes a big bang and it's exciting". Similarly, Tony refers to "the crackling noise and the pops and bangs", which he finds stimulating.

In addition to fire's stimulating properties, participants also make reference to its ability to relax and sedate. For example, Alice says: "it's really comfortable and homely and warm and nice" and Laura says interacting with fire makes her feel "sleepy". This sentiment is echoed repeatedly by my participants, for example, Milly reflects on a coal fire at her family home saying: "it would give me warmth and light in the room; it was comforting" and Sherry describes fire as "a comfort blanket". For some participants, the relaxing properties of fire extend from a feeling of comfort to one of safety as Tyrone says: "everything else around me crumbles. But I'm safe next to the fire". Counter-intuitively, whether participants view fire as arousing or sedating is not simply a function of how they use it. We might assume that reckless (criminalised) uses of fire would arouse, whereas non-criminalised fire use might relax but the distinction is not as simple as that. Consider Kimmy (a predominantly non-criminalised user), above, for example, who speaks of lighting a candle at home as a 'pick me up' (i.e. in order to stimulate).

The notion that participants find the sensory aspects of fire appealing has ample support from existing literature. Broadly speaking from an evolutionary perspective, it makes sense that we should be attracted to something that is life-sustaining. Also, there is evidence to suggest that certain aspects of fire might offer neurological, cognitive and physiological benefits (for example, see Lynn, 2014; Rossano, 2007) and this could also explain its appeal. Furthermore, there are reasons why participants are particularly attracted to the *immediacy and transitory* nature of the effects of fire. For example, Wright (2017) explains that natural selection has 'designed' us to seek out short-lived pleasures repeatedly, such as in the case of sexual intercourse, in order to improve our reproductive success (pp. 7–8).

In addition to the sensory impact of fire discussed above, some of my participants speak of fire use as a means of *releasing* pent-up emotions, namely anger. This has support from the general offending literature whereby anger has been implicated in aggression (for example, see Sell, 2011). Viv epitomises the use of fire as a release as she talks here about her emotional state immediately prior to the arson offence which she committed: "I was angry to the point where I didn't know what I was capable of". Likewise, when reflecting on her feelings at the time of setting a fire, Clarissa states "I felt angry and pissed off with them" in relation to the victims of her firesetting.

So far, I have outlined the first of the Transient Emotional State sub-themes – Immediate Gratification. Fire use also has indirect effects on participants' emotional state and this is represented through the second sub-theme – *Mediator*.

Mediator

This sub-theme is so-called to reflect the way in which fire use can *indirectly* affect participants' emotional state. In other words, fire use can evoke a transient change which acts as a mediator and, in turn, impacts on emotional state. In some instances fire use represents a form of escapism for my participants in that they become someone who is powerful, thus having a positive effect on their emotional state. This is perfectly epitomised by Alice as she recalls how she felt when she was fire-walking: "I was somebody... rather than someone who did everything everyone said, and had no personality whatsoever" and, "fire walking made me feel a lot stronger about me. I was somebody; I was a really, really strong and powerful person". Similarly, Harry describes how he became "an absolute rock star" while fire-performing. The notion of a temporary transformation into 'somebody else' could be understood from the literature on the self. Higgins (1987), for example, writes about three domains to the self: (i) the ideal self, (ii) the actual self, and (iii) the ought self. It might be that in the circumstances my participants are describing here, they are shifting from their actual self to their ideal self, albeit temporarily.

Participants who have engaged in criminalised forms of fire use (namely, arson offences and institutional firesetting) also speak of another mediator, problem resolution; which is where they use fire to solve interpersonal problems leading them to feel better. Rory, for example, speaks of fire-related problem solving within the prison environment: "I had to set fire to my cell to get my mental health medication" and this is echoed by Morris who sets fires in prison to attract attention from staff: "there's no other way of getting staff to my cell door". Participants have also resolved problems in the community through their use of fire, for example, Zane, set a fire to end a relationship which he no longer wanted to be in: "by setting that fire I knew we were never gonna get back together. We couldn't be back together" and Ellen helped her sister to escape an abusive relationship: "the only thing I could get him away with was by me setting the fire". Interestingly, it was only the incarcerated participants in my study who discussed fire use as a problem-solving strategy, which broadly aligns with psychological research addressing the link between social problem-solving deficits and crime (Ross & Fabiano, 1985, as cited in Antonowicz & Ross, 2005; McMurran, Fyffe, McCarthy, Duggan & Latham, 2001).

Summary of the Transient Emotional State theme

This theme is concerned with the immediate but transient physiological effect of fire on participants' emotional state. These effects are perceived as positive and, thus, are reinforcing and make it more likely that participants will repeatedly seek opportunities to interact with fire. The remaining CoFUT themes concern longer-lasting effects. These are discussed below.

Sense of Self

Universal to all participants in my study, irrespective of how they use fire, is the sense that fire forms part of who they are; this is captured within the Sense of Self theme. To be clear, this differs from the transient shift in self-state discussed above because it relates to the longer term. Sense of Self is separated into two sub-themes. The first of these refers to how participants define themselves; in other words, their *Identity* and the second is *Self-Esteem*. The two sub-themes are intrinsically linked because how we define ourselves and how we appraise ourselves both contribute to an overall impression of who we are. Each of the sub-themes is discussed below.

Identity

The concept of identity has received a lot of attention in psychological literature and has manifold definitions. Burke and Stets (2009) and Stets and Burke (2014) propose a framework comprising three *types* of identity: (i) *role*: the social position we consider ourselves to hold, for example, we may view ourselves as a student, or a parent; (ii) *social/group*: the way in which we relate to relevant social group/s, such as those of the same ethnicity, and; (iii) *person*: the characteristics which we believe make us unique. These apply well to the current data.

Firstly, for many of my participants, fire acts as a reminder of their roots. This is an example of person identity (Burke & Stets, 2009; Stets & Burke, 2014) and is exemplified here by Mary: "there's this smell of a peat fire; it's in my bones; I love it. From a time when I was very little". Likewise, Tony and Nelly describe how fire formed an integral part of their early living environment: "on the estate where I lived there'd be empty houses or cars on fire or there'd be a fire built" and "it's a rough estate; there's certain people that are clowns and set people's cars on fire".

Secondly, participants consider themselves to have a fire-related role, which aligns well with another aspect of the framework (Burke & Stets, 2009; Stets & Burke, 2014). Jim, for example, whose role is to light the fire within the family home is meticulous and experienced with the task:

> I take an old newspaper, screw up some sheets into balls, stuff them at the bottom, and then away we go with a match. Usually, if it's nice, and dry material, there's no problem.

Like Jim, Mary also has a fire-related role in the family. She discusses the part she plays in the aftermath of a campfire:

> I'm actually quite neurotic. So if we have a fire in the woods I bring a shovel, and lift the sod. I take the grass off. So we leave it as we found it. That is my training.

Thirdly, fire use also contributes to identity through offering a sense of belonging and togetherness, which helps participants to establish a 'position' in their community or family – this relates to the social/group identity (Burke & Stets, 2009; Stets & Burke, 2014). Jane speaks of the social aspect of communal fires and how it helps her to relate to like-minded people:

> We burn stuff on the fire, have barbeques, and do our fire toys. I guess I've met my fire kindred spirits. Everyone I know likes setting stuff on fire. Everyone likes a good fire.

Likewise, Nelly speaks here of cooperation within her family when preparing a fire: "we're all there together as a family…me and my brothers carry big logs together". This is echoed by Clarissa who attended bonfires at her care home as a child and reflects that she felt "part of something". Some participants even speak of 'connections' on a more existential level, for example, Kimmy describes how the practice of meditating with candles unites her with the universe:

> The flame comes, and then it joins with the air. And so whatever energy and thoughts you're putting to that flame as you focus, it then goes up to the universe. So it's almost like the flame is taking your thought and your prayers up there to the universe.

In the CoFUT there is a conceptual link between Identity, i.e. how participants define themselves, and the second Sense of Self sub-theme entitled Self-Esteem.

Self-Esteem

All of my participants speak of the positive impact of fire use on self-esteem, which is defined as "the positive or negative overall evaluation we have of ourselves" (Gilovich, Keltner & Nisbett, 2010, p. 91). There are a number of routes through which fire use inflates participants' self-esteem according to the data. Whilst this occurs relatively fleetingly it has a cumulative effect, thus, leading to longer term benefits. Firstly, participants gain *external recognition* from others, most often in the form of praise. This is depicted by Alice as she reflects on her fire walk: "it's good because everybody's cheering, and the music's going, and it's really good". Laura echoes this in her reflections as a fire performer: "it's really exciting cause it can make people scream, and it's a good way of getting their attention". Likewise, both Tony and Zane gained kudos from friends through behaving recklessly in their youth. They both speak here of jumping through fire in the presence of friends: "it's something that is between you and your friends; who got the closest to the fire. It's bragging rights" and "it's a male bravado thing". Similarly, Tyrone recalls setting fires as a youth because it made him "look cool".

Participants not only gain self-esteem through impressing their peers with fire use, but also through feeling that they have done a 'good job'. Milly and Sherry, for instance, reflect on building and maintaining fires in the family home when they were young: "I were chuffed because it would give me warmth and light in the room" and "it felt good cause I liked to help; I felt appreciated". Likewise, For Amanda, the ability to maintain a fire is an important benchmark against which she judges herself:

> *I think I do rate myself on making a good fire. Cause I think that's the bit I enjoy; of feeling I've done a good fire; made a proper fire. So, feeling a sense of pride on that front.*

Harry also gains intrinsic value from fire. He reflects here on the long process of practising a particular fire-performing trick and then eventually being able to do it:

> *Then I did it, and I could do it, and lit it, and I was doing this trick on fire. I was doing this trick on fire. It was a life changing moment.*

The crux of the boost to self-esteem which participants speak of is the subjective sense that they can control fire in some way and this seems to impact favourably on their self-esteem. This control is predicated on the ability to manipulate fire to behave as one intends as Mary alludes to here:

> *We have an open fire in the house and we have one of those big square fireguards.*
> *I have a grandson now and it just means that he can play in the room and it's*
> *relatively safe, not absolutely, but relatively safe.*

Similarly, Rory, who was a chef in the past and also has an arson conviction, says: "I've been kitchen manager in places and I've tried to put measures in place so fires don't happen" and Laura, a fire performer, says: "you can get a bit blasé about the level of control that you have over the fire; that can come back to bite you".

The desire to have control over fire makes sense in an evolutionary sense because of its essential role in our survival (Clark & Harris, 1985; Goudsblom, 1992; Pyne, 1998; Wrangham, 2010; Wrangham & Carmody, 2010), as discussed in Chapter 2. However fire, by its very nature, is unpredictable and so, arguably, any interaction with it carries a degree of risk and, thus, a degree of uncertainty. For this reason, I suggest that any perception of control over a fire is subjective; this is supported by Lyng (1990) who refers to "the illusion of control" in risk-taking behaviour (p. 873). I propose within the CoFUT that it is this *subjective* experience of control which feeds into participants' self-esteem.

In his writings on risk-taking, Lyng (1990, 2005) introduces the concept of *edgework,* i.e. the idea that risk-takers, such as sky-divers or rock-climbers, operate by maintaining control whilst on the cusp of chaos. Central to edgework is physical skill but also an ability to overcome emotions such as fear and nervousness. Despite being on the 'brink' edge workers manage to maintain order (Lyng, 1990, p. 871), or, at least, they believe they do. Edgework applies particularly well to my fire performer participants who demonstrate a high degree of skill in remaining in control of a fire prop which could easily cause them significant harm if something went wrong. The potential for this harm is captured here, by Connor, who speaks of the dangers involved: "a female fire performer had a costume related accident and her costume melted to her and she died". He goes on to say:

> *Fire performers tend to be quite blasé – 'it won't hurt me, I'm used to it'. But it's*
> *a big shock to the system when something like that happens that someone who's*
> *so experienced and so well-known has a fatal accident. I've had friends who've set*
> *themselves on fire before; I've set myself on fire before. I know a girl who had a*
> *nasty accident while fire breathing and nearly died. Her lungs started to fill with*
> *fluid and she nearly drowned, which is ironic; fire can make you drown.*

Similarly, edgework can also apply to criminalised forms of fire use. Despite the fact that their behaviour is maladaptive and sometimes, law-breaking, criminalised fire users are arguably still executing a degree of skill because of the dangerousness of the activity. Relating this discussion back to the CoFUT, I am suggesting here that the subjective sense that one is maintaining control in a risky situation is the source of self-esteem.

Summary of the Sense of Self theme

The Sense of Self theme exemplifies how fire use is intertwined with one's identity. It gives participants a sense of purpose, helps them to connect with others and, in some cases, reminds them of their roots. Fire use also aids self-esteem both intrinsically, through having pride in one's fire use, but also extrinsically, through gaining praise from one's peers. In the CoFUT, Sense of Self feeds into the last theme – Psychological Wellbeing.

Psychological Wellbeing

This theme relates to the long-term impact of fire use on participants' psychological wellbeing. It differs from the first CoFUT theme (Transient Emotional State) because it reflects participants' long-standing psychological and mental health, whereas the former is concerned only with short-term and fluid emotional state. In fact, the two themes (Transient Emotional State and Psychological Wellbeing) can be mutually exclusive. It is possible, for example, for someone who is psychologically healthy to be in a temporary state of sadness and, likewise, it is possible for someone who is psychologically unwell to feel happy in specific situations.

The Psychological Wellbeing theme demonstrates how the long-term impact of fire use can vary as a function of the type of relationship a person has formed with it. In other words, data from my study indicate that fire-setting offences and institutional firesetting (i.e. fire use sitting at the criminalised end of the spectrum) have a detrimental impact on psychological wellbeing, whereas that which sits closer to the non-criminalised end (and has, thus, not been reprimanded) promotes psychological health. This variation is reflected in the two sub-themes, the first of which is entitled *Security*, which relates primarily to non-criminalised forms of fire use. It is important to note here that all participants shared examples of non-criminalised fire use occurring at some point in their life, even those with arson convictions. However, examples of the Security sub-theme mainly feature in the narratives of participants engaging *only* in non-criminalised forms of fire use; the sub-theme refers to deeper-rooted *long-term* psychological benefits. When discussing the long-term, the imprisoned participants tend to focus on the drawbacks of the reprimands they have received for criminalised fire use. These drawbacks are depicted by the second sub-theme – *Self-Preservation*.

Security

This sub-theme relates to how the positive characteristics of fire offer a deep and long-lasting sense of security, even when times are hard, and this impacts favourably on psychological health. This is aptly conveyed by George who says:

> *Nurture and warmth and protection. It's in that simplest form that fire warms you and it cooks you food and it makes you tools. So it's at the heart of what keeps you safe and what keeps you alive in a way that most modern people probably don't realise or see, you know.*

This sub-theme concerns the interlinking qualities of fire, which participants consider it to embody, including: (i) inspiration, empowerment and hope; (ii) simplicity and authenticity; (iii) constancy and predictability, and; (iv) companionship, nurturance and protection. A common trend in how participants convey these characteristics is that they personify fire, i.e. they ascribe to it human-like features, as if it has a personality of its own. Ultimately, all of these positive qualities offer a sense of security for participants, which impacts favourably on their overall psychological wellbeing in the long term. Each quality is reviewed below.

Firstly, participants speak of fire's inspirational and empowering properties, alongside it being a representation of hope and this supports participants in their personal growth. For Elle fire even serves as a sort of mentor: "the fire is there to teach you everything you need to know. So the fire becomes a bit of a master; you will see the fire as your guru". Furthermore, many participants speak of the optimism, hope and energy which fire embodies. George, who is a Pagan, conveys hope in this way: "at the heart of that festival for us is a log, and a bright burning fire so that at the darkest part of the year, there's hope". The symbolic meanings ascribed to fire by participants in my study are not surprising given what was discussed in Chapter 2 in reference to the many symbolic representations of fire. For instance, Fessler (2006) calls it a "romanticised marker of special occasions" (p. 441) and Winder (2009) refers to a spiritual appreciation of fire, and suggests that burning a candle is associated with purity, hope, protection and renewal (p. 13).

Another characteristic associated with the Security sub-theme is the simplicity and authenticity of fire, as Amanda explains: "fire just feels quite natural; it's going back to the natural elements side of things. That feels quite nice". Similarly, George recalls situations in his life where he had no access to electricity and so had to rely on fire to meet his basic needs: "there was something rather nice about the fact that we had no electricity, therefore we had none of the distractions of modern life". In addition, many participants also find the constancy of fire to be reassuring, as conveyed by Alice: "it keeps coming back. Fire's gone on forever. You know; fire's gone on forever and the Phoenix rises out of the flames; rebirth and death". The same sentiments are echoed by George who says:

> There's a sense of continuity with fires; the notion of continuity, of life, and of the home as it were. So the common focal point of the fire is the same as the focal point of the fire when a family were living in this house 300 years ago. So that's kind of important, so there's a continuity of human experience that the fire brings out.

In addition to the positive characteristics already outlined above, participants also speak of fire as the embodiment of companionship, nurturance and protection which, in turn, provides a sense of security and peace. This is particularly pertinent in situations where they may otherwise feel uneasy, such as if they are alone, or when they are feeling low. For Mary, for example, fire provides her with company:

> It's one of the comforts I have when I'm in the house by myself. In a way that central heating wouldn't give to me; I do think there's life in fire and company in it.

Here Mary is personifying fire and, thus, it has a similar effect as would a human companion. Similarly, she conveys a sense of comfort in the idea that fire indicates others are close by. When speaking of childhood memories of her neighbours' homes, she says: "in the houses that were near enough to see you'd actually know by the chimney smoke if someone was at home".

For some participants, like Kimmy, fire is also ascribed the human characteristics of caring and nurturing, for example "to me it's nurturing. Certainly if I'm lighting my candle for that end- of-the-day warming, nurturing feeling. That blanket around you and homely feeling". Similarly, Elle says "the fire comes to hug you and the fire brings flowers and everything else. It's a unique thing. You feel a lot of love". Interestingly, Jane uses very similar language when describing fire: "it's like a little hug experience". In addition to companionship and nurturance, some participants speak of fire's protective nature. For example, Connor says:

> You can see what's near the fire and you can't see what's away from it. So away from the fire is where the potential danger lurks and near the fire – in the light and warmth and security of other people – that's where the safety is.

In the CoFUT the sense of security gleaned from fire use relates to feeling peaceful and happy, which aligns with at least two human goods in the Good Lives Model (GLM; Ward & Brown, 2004, p. 247), and thus has clinical implications, returned to in the following chapters. The security associated with non-criminalised forms of fire use could conceivably be traced back to fire's roles in sustaining life, such as through providing warmth and light (Karkanas et al., 2007), enabling us to cook food and produce tools (Fessler, 2006; Wrangham, 2010), offering protection (Clarke & Harris, 1985) and facilitating deep sleep (Wrangham, 2010). That being said, we cannot ignore the fact that we, in the UK at least, also associate fire with danger and negative consequences. For example, Yin (2016) highlights that smoke can burn our eyes and sear our lungs. Also, food could be coated in char, which can increase the risk of cancer. Furthermore, fire encourages people to congregate which could increase the spread of disease. Curiously, however, participants appear able to reconcile these downsides in favour of the benefits. Perhaps this is because of its omnipotence in keeping us alive (recall, for instance, the discussion on the sun in Chapter 2).

In the CoFUT, security is most strongly associated with non-criminalised forms of fire use. Conversely, the most severe forms of criminalised use are associated with long-term psychological damage – this is captured in the next sub-theme entitled *Self-Preservation*.

Self-Preservation

For those participants whose fire use has been reprimanded, there are long-term negative consequences which threaten psychological wellbeing. The psychological harm seems to be coming from their perceived social status as an arsonist/firesetter, as conveyed here by Sherry who has an arson conviction: "it's a stigma – who's gonna trust a person if they have been convicted of arson"? Being 'labelled' in this way impacts detrimentally one's self-esteem. This highlights a partial overlap with the Self-Esteem sub-theme discussed earlier but the current sub-theme relates to a myriad of psychological harms including damage to relationships and quality of life, the blocking of goals for the future and a lack of physical and emotional freedom. In order to mitigate the effects of being labelled, participants employ cognitive self-preservation strategies, which are expounded below. These are akin to similar concepts in the existing psychological and sociological literature, including *mechanisms of defence* (Freud, 2018, p. 42), *cognitive distortions* (Ward, Hudson, Johnston & Marshall, 1997; p. 498), and *neutralisation* (Sykes & Matza, 1957, p. 666).

The way that participants utilise self-preservation could be conceptualised as a repetitive 'push-pull' cognitive process. Being labelled threatens psychological health and so the use of self-preservation strategies becomes a way of coping. It is possible that, over time, these strategies could lead to the formation of a new self-narrative for that person, i.e. a permanent change in how they view their criminal past. This is akin to a process which Maruna (2001) has written extensively about called *narrative repair*. According to Maruna, *redemptive narratives* are a means of correcting the stigmatisation suffered on account of having committed a crime. This can actually lead to changes in particular aspects of the person's identity from 'anti-social' to 'pro-social', which have been found to play a role in desistance (Maruna, 2001; Rocque, Posick & Paternoster, 2016). In reporting on the Liverpool Desistance Study, Maruna (2001) identifies five types of redemptive narrative, a number of which are reminiscent of my participants' self-preservation strategies as outlined below.

One of the self-preservation strategies identified in the data is where participants try to self-affirm that firesetting holds no residual temptation to them and, thus, that they no longer pose a risk. For example, Milly says: "arson is something that I won't be doing again", Zane says: "I will never ever – whether people believe it or not – I will never ever set fire to anything ever again", and Morris says: "as time's gone on I've lost interest in firesetting". Similarly, Tony says "if I see a car on fire now I wouldn't give it two thoughts. I'd walk past it; I wouldn't even give it a second glance". Additionally, participants state their dislike, hatred and mistrust of fire as a whole entity, thus further affirming that they have no desire to be near to it again. For example, Rory says: "fire is the enemy. That's what I've come to think now", which is echoed by Tia: "fire is evil in disguise; it's like the devil. It comes in many forms, like evil". Sherry speaks more directly about the dangers of fire: "it can kill people. Or leave them badly scarred. It can destroy families and friendships", as does Zane: "it's a killer. It can kill people". There are similarities between the way in which participants think of fire here and one of the redemptive scripts identified in the Liverpool Desistance Study (LDS; Maruna, 2001). Participants in the LDS speak of a bad 'it', i.e. something external to themselves which might be responsible for their past criminal behaviour. In this case, the bad 'it' is fire.

Another self-preservation strategy featuring in participants' narratives is the process of mentally distancing oneself from one's behaviour; this comes in a number of forms. First, participants deny and/or seek to excuse aspects of their criminalised fire use. For example, Sherry minimises her motivation for committing the arson offence: "I really didn't do it intending to harm someone" and Rory adopts a victim stance: "what did I get for my troubles? It's led me into a life of being in prison". Some participants also seek to minimise their actions, for example, Zane says: "I'm gonna be labelled now as an arsonist. Yes, I've committed an arson attack but I'm not an arsonist. I didn't get no excitement from it. I wasn't happy about it". Similarly, Clarissa says: "I've never actually set a house on fire. I wouldn't because that's going over the top". Secondly, some participants appear to adopt an 'advocate' role, i.e. to speak on behalf of others and to promote fire safety. Rory, for example, says that fire-related deaths are "something that the government needs to look at" and Sherry alludes here to the importance of education relating to fire safety: "when you're lighting a fire you're not thinking about where the smoke's going. And how it's gonna affect other people. It's lack of education". The notion of adopting an advocacy role and seeking to improve fire safety for others is reminiscent of another of the redemptive scripts highlighted in the LDS (Maruna, 2001). Maruna's participants speak of positive futures through making a commitment to developing people.

According to the Self-Preservation sub-theme, being labelled an arsonist/fire-setter is psychologically harmful. Why, then, have the imprisoned participants in my study continued to engage in criminalised fire use? As outlined above, the self-preservation strategies act as a buffer but there might also be other mechanisms at play. I propose that the allure of the immediate gains from fire (i.e. as described in the Transient Emotional State theme) is so great that it might override the negatives of being stigmatised. The pull of these immediate gains might be particularly strong for some because of deficits in self-control, which have been found to be predictive of crime (see Mears, Cochran & Beaver, 2013).

Summary of the Psychological Wellbeing theme

This theme relates to the long-term impact of fire use on participants' psychological wellbeing. It demonstrates how the long-term impact of fire use can vary as a function of the type of relationship a person has formed with it. In other words, data indicate that firesetting offences and institutional firesetting (i.e. fire use sitting at the criminalised end of the spectrum) have a detrimental impact on psychological wellbeing, whereas that which sits closer to the non-criminalised end (and has not been reprimanded) has a positive effect.

Application

Any new theory, such as the CoFUT outlined in this chapter, should be evaluated. In other words, how good is the theory? How useful is it? Is it consistent with existing literature? Above, I highlighted support for the CoFUT's constituent themes from the existing literature. Finding support, in the form of existing theory and research, is an important aspect of what makes a 'good' theory, which Ward and Beech (2006) refer to as *external consistency* (p. 46). Another important point for evaluation is to consider the *utility* of a theory or what Ward and Hudson refer to as *fertility or heuristic value* (p. 46). In other words, can it be usefully and meaningfully applied in a forensic setting, such as a prison or hospital by forensic practitioners like psychologists, probation officers and mental health professionals? In the next two chapters I will outline how the CoFU as a broad conceptualisation and the CoFUT, specifically, can be used as a basis for assessment and treatment with those who set fires. These discussions will demonstrate, I argue, that the CoFUT has fertility/heuristic value. Before moving on to discuss how the theory can guide practice more generally, however, I will discuss how it could be applied, specifically, to cases where people have set fires. To do this I will draw upon two service users with whom I have worked as a practitioner in order to highlight how the CoFUT can be applied. It is important to emphasise that the service users' names have been changed, as has any other identifiable information, such as age. The discussions below are deliberately broad in order to protect the service users' anonymity, for example, I have not provided specific details about their index offences.

Mike

Mike is 34 and is convicted of arson. He was serving a prison sentence when I was asked to conduct a risk assessment with him for the purpose of a parole review. In an interview with Mike, I asked him to recall experiences of fire use in his early life. He responded, initially, by telling me that he had no such memories and denied that fire played any part in his life prior to adulthood. In my experience, this is typically a service user's first response to the question. However, after giving them some time to consider their past, they often start to remember more information, albeit they might not necessarily see the relevance of it initially. In our second interview, Mike informed me that he had been thinking about the question I posed and that, in fact, he had started to recall a series of "fire memories".

Mike's early home life was unstable and volatile; he fought with his siblings and he described emotionally neglectful parents. Despite this, he told me that his father would regularly light fires in the garden in order to dispose of household and garden waste. Mike remembers those times as being very positive and described his whole family congregating around the fire, talking, laughing and telling stories. He recalled an image of seeing the "bright sparks" float into the air, contrasting with the dark night sky. Here, he was discussing a visual element of fire, which is an example of immediate gratification – a part of the Transient Emotional State theme in the CoFUT. There were also other examples of immediate gratification in Mike's case in the form of sensory stimulation. He told me of times that he would set fire to toys in order to watch the flames melt the plastic and to enjoy the smell it would produce. Furthermore, he told me he would often play with his mother's cigarette lighter because he enjoyed watching the flames. Interestingly, there was also evidence of a 'release' of pent-up emotions in Mike's case; in reference to the index offence he explained to me that he was "angry" and wanted to seek "revenge" on his victim. This release of emotions is also of relevance to the Immediate Gratification sub-theme, as discussed above.

When speaking of family time in the garden, Mike remembered assisting his father with the building and maintenance of the fire, which he felt was a source of attention from his father. Mike's recollection of being together as a family, in addition to helping out with fire-related tasks aligns well with the Sense of Self theme in the CoFUT, particularly the Self-Esteem sub-theme. In my contact with Mike, he spoke of the detrimental impact, which the prison sentence has had on his mental health. He told me that he regrets his actions and "never [has] urges to set fires" any longer; these statements are examples of the self-preservation strategies which form part of the Psychological Wellbeing CoFUT theme.

Greg

Greg is 30 and is serving a prison sentence for arson. He has two previous arson convictions on record and also self-reported a number of incidents, which would conceivably be seen as sitting towards the criminalised end of the CoFU. Greg's earliest memory of fire was enjoying the coal fire within his foster parents' home. He recalled his foster parents' lighting this on winter days. He relayed memories of the "crackling" sound and of watching the different colours of the flames, which he described as "red, yellow, green… dancing around". The stimulating features of fire which Greg was referring to here align well with the Immediate Gratification sub-theme within the CoFUT. Similarly, he also made reference to the "cosy" and relaxing aspects of fire which are another example of immediate gratification. Greg recalled "family nights" in front of the fire as they watched television, which he told me made him feel "safe". There is a sense of togetherness here, which aligns with the Sense of Self theme. Furthermore, the safety he speaks of is reminiscent of the Psychological Wellbeing sub-theme – Security, which is mostly associated with non-criminalised forms of fire use in the CoFUT.

In contrast, Greg reflected on the detrimental impact of his imprisonment for the (index) arson offence. Like Mike, he explained to me that his time in prison has resulted in deterioration of his mental health, including paranoia and anxiety. Greg told me that he hated himself and needs help with his mental health particularly. He also emphasised that he would never deliberately harm another person and he regrets his offences. In my assessment of him, I also noted instances of victim blaming; these are examples of self-preservation as discussed within the CoFUT.

Evaluation and future directions

In presenting the CoFUT, I do not assert that this is the 'finished product'. In the spirit of grounded theory (the method employed in my research, see Horsley, 2020), I intend to collect more data, which will lead to revisions and extensions being made. The CoFUT, and the data on which it is based are not without limitations, a detailed appraisal of which is provided in Horsley (2020). For example, sampling bias might explain the significance that fire users in my study place on fire; I deliberately sought to speak to people who use fire extensively and, thus, this might explain why it is such an important part of their sense of self and psychological wellbeing. It is possible that less frequent fire users might view it very differently. Similar studies should be conducted with a broader range of people to explore whether the CoFUT still applies. That being said, I have already supervised one such study at the Master's level in my academic role. A study by Lee (2019) explored the experiences and views of what we termed 'moderate' fire users, namely people who have infrequent contact with fire and for whom it does not play any particular overt role in their life. It is significant to note that Lee identified very similar themes in her data. For example, a theme entitled Self Concept was identified, which is very similar to Sense of Self in the CoFUT. This suggests that even for people who do not choose to interact with fire often, it still plays a part in their impression of who they are.

In this chapter, I have already addressed two of the characteristics which Ward and Beech (2006) consider to make a 'good' theory (p. 46), namely, external consistency and fertility/heuristic value. Ward and Beech also discuss other characteristics such as simplicity, which they define as making "the fewest theoretical assumptions" (p. 46). I assert that the CoFUT achieves this in that it is grounded in the data from my study and there are no 'assumptions' beyond that, apart from references to mechanisms such as reinforcement, which already feature widely in the firesetting literature.

There are other aspects of a 'good' theory which I accept that the CoFUT has not fully accomplished, such as explanatory depth, defined as the "theory's ability to describe deep underlying causes and processes" (p. 46). The detail I have provided in describing the CoFUT sub-themes goes some way to achieving depth. For example, in relation to the Self-Esteem sub-theme, I provided detail on the different forms that this can take for participants, such as personal pride and external recognition. Similarly, in commenting on the Self-Preservation sub-theme, I elaborated on the different types of strategies participants employ. Notwithstanding these details, more research is required to refine the CoFUT and to develop its explanatory depth. Importantly, I am not claiming that the CoFUT, with any certainty, can be generalised to *all* fire users. It is, after all, based on one qualitative study. That being said, there is some debate about whether generalisability should be a meaningful goal for qualitative research at all (Braun & Clarke, 2013, p. 280).

In considering generalisability further, I agree with the view of Yardley (2008, as cited in Braun & Clarke, 2013, p. 281) who states "there is little point in doing research if every situation was totally unique, and the results in one study had no relevance to any other situation". I think it is entirely reasonable to think that there might be at least some degree of similarity between the fire users in my study and other fire users. I make this claim for a number of reasons. Firstly, there was a high degree of overlap in the narratives of predominantly non-criminalised and predominantly criminalised participants in my study. This points to there being certain core features underpinning the human-fire relationship irrespective of the *type* of fire use, which, in turn supports the dimensional argument. Secondly, I have demonstrated external consistency by highlighting where my findings are supported by existing theory and research. Thirdly, in my practitioner experience, there are clinical cases where the CoFUT can be applied as exemplified above, which is a preliminary indicator of clinical utility.

Summary

Grounded in the data from 24 participants, the CoFUT comprises three themes which depict the psychological impact of fire use and, more broadly, psychological features of the human-fire relationship. Importantly, these themes are common to a wide range of fire uses thereby supporting the argument for a dimensional conceptualisation. The CoFUT advances existing knowledge through offering a holistic perspective on the human-fire relationship, rather than solely seeking to explain firesetting or arson. The CoFUT is only in its preliminary stages of development but I argue it already has clinical utility. Understanding fire use in this way, alongside a broader consideration of how it is socially constructed, as well as its importance in the evolution and survival of our species, is of crucial importance in advancing assessment, treatment and intervention. This will be the focus of the following two chapters.

Assessing people who set fires

6

A holistic approach

Overview

There are no existing risk assessment tools specifically designed for those who light fires (Watt & Ong, 2016), which has traditionally resulted in a 'one size fits all' approach. In fact, as a practitioner, whilst I have observed progress in the treatment of people who set fires (discussed in the next chapter), I have not seen the same steps in assessment and so this urgently requires attention. It is important to note at this point that in discussing assessment, I will refer specifically to the work of forensic psychologists to reflect my own professional background but much of what is discussed here can also apply to allied forensic practitioners to include the work of probation services and healthcare professionals. I argue that, historically, the approach we have taken in the assessment of people who set fires has been too narrow and that we should be seeking to see the bigger picture. I suggest that utilising the term fire *use*, rather than firesetting is a sensible starting point. In this chapter, I will highlight some of the issues with the existing approach to assessment and propose how we can move practice forward. I will also include examples of best practice. Before turning to these matters, however, it is important to provide some context on the type of assessments undertaken by forensic psychologists and allied professionals.

Forensic assessment

In conducting assessments, forensic psychologists and allied professionals are often tasked with assessing the reasons behind an offence and the risk with which

DOI: 10.4324/9780367808648-6

a service user presents, as well as their treatment needs and readiness (Brown, Shell & Cole, 2015, p. 258). It is worth noting here that risk encompasses many nuanced considerations including the nature and level of risk, alongside how it can be best managed (Brown et al., 2015, p. 258) – this is returned to below. For the current purpose, we can broadly think of risk as being the likelihood of a service user re-offending and, if they did, what this offence might look like and the level of harm it might cause to others.

A good forensic risk assessment should incorporate a case formulation which aids understanding of the service user's offending behaviour. In brief, formulation is defined as "a provisional explanation or hypothesis of how an individual comes to present with a certain disorder or circumstance at a particular point in time" (Weerasekera, 1996, as cited in Dallos, Stedmon & Johnstone, 2014, p. 181). In forensic assessment, the 'circumstance' could be the index offence. In developing a formulation, forensic practitioners typically include reference to predisposing (i.e. background) factors and precipitants to the offence (Dudley & Kuyken, 2014). In the case of firesetting specifically, I suggest that predisposing factors should include consideration of the person's lifelong relationship with fire. Precipitating factors should include triggers to the firesetting and can be gleaned through an analysis of the offence itself in order to explore how it came about. This can be helpful in illuminating the function/s of the crime. I suggest this could be structured around the different stages of fire use which are outlined below. It is worth noting here that the best case formulations are collaborative; the service user should have the opportunity to contribute and to comment on whether they believe the finished product provides an accurate picture of who they are and their offending behaviour.

This chapter is structured in line with the aforementioned broad formulation framework, starting with the assessment of predisposing factors. This should include holistically understanding a service user's lifelong relationship with fire, as well as other pertinent features of their background history. This will be followed by some discussion on precipitants and the offence analysis and lastly, risk monitoring and management considerations.

Predisposing factors

Fire use history

In Chapter 4, I discussed literature on positive psychology (for reviews, see Seligman & Csikszentmihalyi, 2000; Seligman, Steen, Park & Peterson, 2005) and how this is starting to pervade forensic research and practice (for discussions, see Towl & Crighton, 1996; Ward, 2017). Despite the persuasiveness of the argument for a more positive take on working with forensic service users in my experience it has not yet fully been translated into changes in practice. Terms such as *risk, risk factor* and *risk assessment* are still commonplace in a forensic psychologist's vernacular, which is likely the result of the historic emphasis on these factors in the psychological literature (for examples, see Whitaker et al., 2008; Mann, Hanson & Thornton, 2010; Farrington, Gaffney & Ttofi, 2017) rather than the more contemporary protective factors (for examples, see de Vogel, de Vries Robbé, de Ruiter & Bouman, 2011; De Vries Robbé, Mann, Maruna & Thornton, 2015). Nevertheless, a shift is happening, and this is highly relevant to practitioners' work with those who light fires. As discussed previously, the continuum of fire use (CoFU) conceptualisation aligns closely with principles of positive psychology. It promotes a way of thinking about the human-fire relationship, which, could be applied in the assessment of those who light fires. I suggest that the CoFU could provide a framework for clinicians to explore the full range of a service user's fire history and that this is a key predisposing factor.

In Chapter 5, I outlined examples of how the participants in my qualitative study (Horsley, 2020) used fire in the following list:

- Functional use – cooking food over fire, the use of fire to keep warm or to complete a task, such as welding;
- Recreational use – this broad category comprises the lighting of bonfires, campfires, candles, fireworks, coal fires and log burners all for the primary purpose of enjoyment;
- Vocational use – the use of fire by artists who are paid to entertain with fire, such as fire jugglers and fire breathers;
- Spiritual and ritualistic use – rituals and ceremonies, for example, the use of fire to cleanse/ward off evil;
- Religious use – the lighting of candles and fires, as well as the burning of objects for religious purposes;
- Self-harm through the use of fire (i.e. by burning one's skin);
- Reckless fire play, including attempts to run through bonfires, aiming fireworks at people and burning objects over a fire (such as childhood toys);
- Setting fire to outdoor public spaces, namely parks/grassland;
- Setting fire to vehicles;
- Setting fire to residential buildings (including houses and flats).

I have arranged the above list in a particular order to reflect where I think these forms of fire use may sit on the CoFU, ranging from non-criminalised (at the top) to criminalised. However, the ordering of this list is subjective, which is reminiscent of the discussion in Chapter 4 on the difficulties in demarcating legal and illegal practices and the "grey areas" in between (Botoeva, 2019; p. 68).

The factors which might influence where one chooses to position types of fire use along the continuum are manifold. As already discussed, I suggest that one of these is cultural background. It is reasonable to assume that if culture influences how we *use* fire (as discussed by Fessler, 2006; Winder, 2009; Ó Ciardha & Gannon, 2012; Horsley, 2020) then it follows that it would influence how we *perceive* fire use as well (Horsley, 2020).

The list above captures only some examples of fire use; there are many more, including those which we might not even think of as fire such as a barbeque, a gas cooker or even gas central heating. Owing to the flame in the boiler. As discussed in Chapter 2, I suggest that in the Global North we take fire for granted because many of us do not come across it in its most primitive form – the naked flame – as frequently as our ancestors would have done. The more we stop to consider fire use in the UK, the more examples we can generate (I am concentrating, here, on the UK because this is where my research has taken place to date). Taking the list above as an example, I suggest that exploring the full continuum of a service user's fire use could contribute to a fuller understanding of how they came to commit fire-related crime. In other words, this can provide an insight into their lifelong relationship with fire.

In assessing fire use, the work of Canter and Fritzon (1998) offers a helpful structure. The authors present a classification system for arson, which I suggest can usefully be applied to fire use more widely. Canter and Fritzon discuss different modes of action in an arson offence, which are a function of both the *target* of the fire (either an object or a person) and the *motivation* behind the offence (either an expressive or an instrumental act). For example, one person might target a residential building for the purpose of destroying evidence of a burglary – this is an instrumental act because it is being perpetrated in pursuit of another goal (i.e. to destroy evidence). Conversely, another person might set fire to themselves in the form of "suicide by arson" for the purpose of relieving emotional distress (p. 75) – this would be considered an expressive motivation (i.e. to express an emotional state).

In assessing those who have set fires, Canter and Fritzon's system could be applied to explore how a service user has used fire in the past - an important predisposing factor. More specifically, they could be asked to identify every type of fire they have used in the past and their motivations for doing so. In my experience this extends beyond current practice, wherein the focus tends only to be on the offence. For instance, in addition to firesetting itself, a service user might report a history of lighting candles to relax, lighting incense burners for religious worship, and using a welding torch for professional duties. All of this is important in understanding their lifelong relationship with fire. Indeed, in my work with people serving prison sentences for firesetting, their non-criminalised experiences often reveal really valuable information. Drawing on the continuum conceptualisation, it could also be helpful to explore the service user's

	Relaxation	Excitement
Candle		
A Person's Home		

Figure 6.1 An extract from the FUM.

perspective on where their fire use sits (i.e. how criminalised they consider it to be); this could provide an insight into their thought process.

Drawing on Canter and Fritzon's system, I have begun developing a tool based on a preliminary pilot study and the existing literature (for example Presdee, 2005; Fessler, 2006; Winder, 2009; Horsley, 2020). This tool - the Fire Use Matrix (FUM) – will include a series of pre-defined fire type/motive combinations such as in the extract in Figure 6.1. The columns along the top of the matrix correspond to motives and the columns down the side correspond to targets. Each cell in the matrix, therefore, corresponds to a particular fire type/motive combination. Through further research I hope to refine this tool and to develop a scoring template in order to calculate a total fire use score. The higher the total score the more criminalised a person's lifetime fire use has been.

The FUM has potential as a research tool, once it has been refined. For example, it could be used to explore the relationship between a person's lifetime fire use (as opposed to just using the firesetter/non-firesetter dichotomy) and a whole host of variables including offence history and psychological characteristics (discussed below). On a more nuanced level, the FUM could be used to explore individual fire use type/motivation combinations and how they relate to the aforementioned variables. For example, research has not yet explored whether, for some people, ostensibly innocuous forms of fire use, such as lighting a candle for relaxation, are, in any way, related to later offending. If we discover that there is a link between particular types of fire use and variables of interest like offence history, fire interest, impulsivity and so on then the FUM could feed into the risk assessment process for those who set fires.

Notwithstanding the FUM's potential as a research tool, it is yet to be refined and validity and reliability would need to be established. In the meantime, I am suggesting that the notion of fire type/ motive combinations, could be applied in the assessment of those who have set fires and could make a valuable contribution to the resultant clinical formulation.

In the discussion above, I have placed an emphasis on fire use history. In work with forensic service users, this could be thought of as a static factor, i.e. something in a person's past which cannot change. Dynamic (i.e. changeable) factors might also serve as predisposers and so are important in the assessment of those who light fires, some of which are reviewed below.

Dynamic considerations

Fire interest and attitudes

A dynamic factor which has attracted the attention of contemporary researchers in the field is fire interest and attitudes. Ó Ciardha et al. (2015a,b) present five 'fire-specific' factors of relevance in the assessment of firesetters, namely:

- Identification with fire – fire as essential to personal identity/functioning;
- Serious fire interest – excitement associated with destructive/life-threatening fires;
- Poor fire safety – a perceived lack of fire safety knowledge;
- Everyday fire interest – excitement associated with non-dangerous normative firesetting scenarios, and;
- Firesetting as normal – views that setting fires is a relatively usual occurrence.

Ó Ciardha et al.'s research indicates that these five factors are of relevance in understanding firesetters' behaviour and should be considered by clinicians who are tasked with assessing firesetters. Furthermore, all but one of the five factors (everyday fire interest) was found to discriminate between firesetters and non-firesetters, albeit in a solely male prison-based sample. With this in mind, practitioners should, at the very least, be considering the four most relevant factors in their assessment of a firesetter to establish whether they hold particular interests and attitudes which might relate to risk. Furthermore, Ó Ciardha et al. (2015a,b) propose that the assessment of these factors is useful in guiding decision-making on the treatment needs of firesetters. This all adds weight to the argument that the 'one size fits all' approach is outdated and insufficient.

Fire-related beliefs

Ó Ciardha et al. (2015b) propose that "future research should attempt to identify whether additional beliefs and attitudes surrounding fire may be criminogenic" beyond the factors outlined above (pp. 45–46). During the course of my doctoral research, through consulting the interdisciplinary literature, as well as drawing on my practitioner experience, I identified a broad framework of additional beliefs which might warrant investigation, both from a clinical and empirical perspective. I have presented these beliefs on three polarities, which were outlined in Chapter 2. To re-cap, these polarities are presented in Figure 6.2.

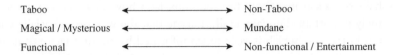

Taboo   ←————————→   Non-Taboo

Magical / Mysterious   ←————————→   Mundane

Functional   ←————————→   Non-functional / Entertainment

Figure 6.2 The three polarities.

In presenting the three polarities I am suggesting that how 'taboo' a person considers fire and fire use to be, alongside how 'magical/mysterious' they view it and the extent to which they see fire as a 'functional' tool are all relevant in the assessment of people who light fires. In support of these points for consideration we can recall the work of Fessler (2006) who highlights that children in a semi-traditional Bengkulu Malay fishing village who were exposed to fire as a functional tool from an early age appeared less interested in playing with it than western children. Conversely, Fessler makes reference to the "strong prohibitions" against childhood fire play in western nations, which might mean that adolescence presents the first opportunity to experiment with fire (p. 438). Likewise, Gannon et al. (2012) refer to the "forbidden" nature of fire, which might serve to increase fire interest (p. 19). It makes sense, then, that the more 'taboo' fire and fire use is considered to be, the more likely people might be to experiment with it, particularly the young. Likewise, the less functionally a person views fire, then the more inclined they are to engage with it for entertainment. This, in turn, overlaps with how magical and mysterious fire is believed to be. From a practical point of view, the three polarities illuminate one central point: that if we teach children only about the dangers of fire and forbid them from interacting with it in mundane circumstances, this might increase intrigue surrounding it. There are parallels here to be drawn with cross-disciplinary research, for example Fisher and Birch (1999) found that when children's access to a palatable food item was restricted by their parents, they were more inclined to seek access to it and to verbalise their desire to consume it.

The three polarities being proposed here are closely intertwined with culture. Unfortunately, whilst cultural considerations underpinning fire use are alluded to in the psychological literature (for examples see Winder, 2009; Gannon et al., 2012) they have never been systematically and empirically addressed. I argue strongly that there is vast cultural variation in the use of fire, with western countries associating it mainly with entertainment and symbolism (Fessler, 2006; Winder, 2009) and less industrialised and/or developed countries having a more pronounced functional reliance on the naked flame (Fessler, 2006). The significance of cultural background in determining how people interact with fire and the types of beliefs they hold is an important theme to explore in future research because this could guide clinical practice in the assessment of those who light fires. Certainly, giving consideration to how cultural background can shape one's learning about fire and, thus, later how they go on to use it, is extremely important. Fundamentally, I argue that the way fire is socially constructed in the UK (which is very much informed by cultural factors) means that it is enshrouded by mystery, intrigue and magic, which might serve only to increase its appeal. Whilst this begins in childhood, it likely continues into adult life. If we could learn more about the influence of culture, particularly in countries where there are lower rates of arson (albeit with the caveat that crime rates are recorded differently from country to country), this could impact on strategy and policy in the UK. This is a novel and, indeed, nuanced topic and so it will take time to develop. The polarities discussed above relate to fire beliefs, which is a dynamic factor in that this can change over time. Other dynamic factors worthy of consideration in the assessment of people who light fires are proposed below.

Sensory stimulation

The mystery with which fire is enshrouded in the UK is, in my view, particularly problematic given its sensory appeal, as evidenced by the Immediate Gratification theme in the CoFUT (see Chapter 5). My research findings (Horsley, 2020) indicate that fire use has a direct effect on one's physiological state and this has also been referred to by others, such as Gannon et al., in the M-TTAF (2012, p. 31). The degree to which one's senses are stimulated in the presence of fire is likely affected by many mediating factors, including culture. For example, owing to novelty, it could be argued that children who are not routinely exposed to fire might find it more appealing from a sensory perspective than those who consider it a normal part of everyday life - a point alluded to by Ó Ciardha and Gannon (2012). In other words, it is possible that people living in countries and specific communities where fire is regularly used primarily as a functional tool have been *de-sensitised* to fire. It is worth noting, however, that the work of Murray et al., (2015) offers a more nuanced perspective - returned to in Chapter 7.

When assessing those with a history of lighting fires, it is prudent to consider the nature of physiological arousal to fire. For example, does the service user report a reduction or increase in their arousal level surrounding fire? My research suggests either can be relevant. Also, it would be helpful for clinicians to establish what aspects of fire, specifically, result in a change in arousal for the service user. Are they particularly attracted to the smell of smoke, the 'crackle' of a burning log, or the sight of the flames? This is important because it could inform treatment targets and the information can feed into risk monitoring and management, for instance, in raising awareness of offence paralleling behaviours (see below).

Fire and sense of self

Data from my research (Horsley, 2020) indicates that for some users, fire is interwoven with identity. This has support from Ó Ciardha et al. (2015b), whose study found that male firesetters are more likely to identify with fire than non-firesetters. Fire use can also impact on a person's self-esteem. In assessing those who set fires; therefore, I recommend that clinicians explore the nature of service users' personal *connection* with fire. This is all part of exploring their lifelong relationship with fire, which should feed into a clinical formulation and, ultimately, contribute to understanding the nature of risk and identifying treatment options. For example, if we determine that criminalised fire use forms part of a service user's sense of self then we have to be aware that simply seeking to 'remove' it could have negative psychological consequences. We can imagine this by considering what contributes to our own sense of self. If, for instance, we identify strongly as a wife or husband, the breakdown of the marriage could leave us feeling incomplete and, thus, impact negatively on our identity and self-esteem. The same applies to service users who desist from crime, if crime has played a significant part in their life until that point. This idea is integral to the strengths-based approach, which advocates that bolstering positive aspect of a service user's life rather than seeking to target 'deficits' is a more productive and compassionate way forward in the rehabilitation of those who have committed crime, as demonstrated through the application of the Good Lives Model (see Ward & Brown, 2004 for an overview).

Once a practitioner has identified key predisposing factors in a service user's life and presentation (both static and dynamic), it is helpful to analyse the fire-related offence specifically.

Precipitating factors and the offence analysis

As well as establishing a service user's fire history, as well as any relevant attitudes and beliefs, it is, of course, still prudent to explore the precipitants to the offence and the offence itself. As already discussed the act of firesetting has been the focus of the vast majority of the existing literature (for examples see Ó Ciardha & Gannon, 2012; Barrowcliffe & Gannon, 2015, 2016). The emphasis here is, thus, on the act of *lighting a fire* as an isolated event. On the contrary, all 24 participants in my own research shared experiences relating to the context surrounding their interactions with fire, the preparation of fires, being in the presence of fire and the aftermath. This supports the idea of a fire use *process,* comprising different stages, and this is partly why I believe that the term fire *use* is more appropriate than firesetting. But, is this not just semantics? Does it really matter? I argue, yes, it does.

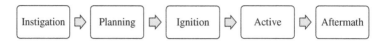

Figure 6.3 The stage model of fire use.

I suggest that it is helpful for forensic practitioners to think of a single instance of fire use (including an offence) as a process, rather than an event, because it could help us to develop a deeper insight into the service user's behaviour and, indeed, the motivations underpinning it.

From my data I identified five stages of fire use (Horsley, 2020) which are depicted in Figure 6.3 and are described as follows: (i) *instigation* which includes experiencing initial thoughts about lighting a fire and considering where and when this might take place; (ii) *planning* which involves taking practical steps in order to organise the fire, namely purchasing and/or collecting materials and building it; (iii) *ignition* is the act of lighting the fire; (iv) the *active* phase occurs while the fire is burning – this can include what the person does to maintain it and their subjective experience of being in the presence of a fire; (v) *aftermath* which involves any post-active behaviour, including extinguishing the fire and cleaning the area. In criminalised fire use this also involves any behaviour undertaken to evade being apprehended.

The findings of my own research offer a novel alternative to the way we think about a single instance of fire use. Typically, a forensic psychological formulation might focus most heavily on the build-up to an offence and the offence itself. This is important and includes consideration of precipitating factors. However, doing this in isolation risks missing important information such as a detailed analysis of the service user's behaviour during the active phase of a fire, as well as how they behaved in the aftermath. I suggest, therefore, that systematic consideration of the five stages described above could elicit a fuller understanding of a service user's behaviour which, in turn, results in a more detailed formulation. This could be further informed by offence chain theories (Tyler, Gannon, Lockerbie, King, Dickens & De Burca, 2014; Barnoux, Gannon & Ó Ciardha, 2015). Breaking down an instance of fire use, including a firesetting offence, can aid the practitioner in planning an interview session. Examples of useful questions for the interview are provided in Table 6.1.

I suggest that structuring an offence account session around the five stages of fire use could be helpful for practitioners. Understanding the wider context surrounding an instance of firesetting is conducive to developing a detailed formulation. We might discover pertinent information by exploring the active stage in detail; for instance, we could detect references to sensory stimulation and its effects. Similarly, the service user's actions in the aftermath might be very revealing, such as how, why and when they came to extinguish the fire where applicable.

Table 6.1 Fire Use Process Questions

Stage	Questions
Instigation	When did you first think about setting a fire and why? Did you consider other options? If so, why were these discounted? What was your objective? How did you decide how and when to set the fire?
Planning	How did you prepare for setting the fire? What materials did you acquire and from where? Tell me about what you did at the scene before the fire was lit.
Ignition	How did you light the fire (e.g. was incendiary fluid used)? What were your thoughts as you lit the fire? How did you feel as the fire took hold?
Active	What did you do once the fire was burning (i.e. remained at scene or fled)? *If remained at the scene:* Why? What did you do while the fire was burning? What did you notice about the fire? Was there anything that you liked/disliked about it? [Professional should probe sensory aspects of fire such as smell, aesthetics and sounds]. How did you feel/what did you think as the fire burned? *If emergency services arrived whilst still at the scene:* How did you feel/ what did you think when the emergency services arrived? Was there anything you noticed (i.e. does the service user discuss their liking of fire engines, etc.)?
Aftermath	How was the fire extinguished? Why did you extinguish the fire when you did? How did you feel/what did you feel once the fire had gone out? What did you do afterwards? (e.g. any evidence of cleaning the area) *If service user extinguished the fire:* Why did you extinguish the fire/how did you decide *when* to extinguish it? How did you extinguish the fire?

Risk monitoring and management

As well as formulating a service user's offence, the risk assessment process should involve supervising and monitoring them and devising a dynamic risk management plan. Information can be gleaned through the way in which a service user presents in custody. Below, two considerations are outlined, which could be of use in developing risk management plans.

Self-preservation strategies

As outlined in the CoFUT the convicted participants in my study (Horsley, 2020) made statements akin to what have been described as cognitive distortions in the sexual offending literature (for examples, see Blumenthal, Gudjonsson & Burns, 1999; Howitt & Sheldon, 2007; Pervan & Hunter, 2007). I conceptualise these statements as self-preservation strategies in that they have aided my participants in the re-writing of their life narrative, thus, mitigating the psychological threat of the stigma attached to being a convicted firesetter. I suggest that there is great value in exploring these strategies when assessing and monitoring those who light fires, particularly their function. However, I will discuss in the following chapter that the negation of these self-preservation strategies should not necessarily be a treatment target per se.

Risk paralleling behaviour

Through my work with people who have firesetting histories I have become familiar with behaviour which may indicate ongoing interest in, or attraction to, fire. Clinical observation of this behaviour is crucial in ensuring effective risk management and, indeed, in being aware of any reduction of risk and relevant protective factors. Many of these behaviours are nuanced and yet are highly relevant for those monitoring a service user's presentation in prison or hospital. As mentioned above, those who light fires might be attracted to particular aspects of fire, such as the colour of the flame or the smell of smoke. In secure settings they are unlikely to have much opportunity to interact with fire, but this does not, necessarily, mean that its appeal has lessened. In the absence of direct contact with fire, it is prudent for forensic practitioners to be aware of subtle behaviours which could mirror interactions with fire. Offence paralleling behaviour (OPB) is defined as "any form of offence related behavioural (or fantasized behaviour) pattern that emerges at any point... [that resembles], in some significant respect, the sequence of behaviours leading up to the offence" (Jones, 2004; p. 38). Jones is explaining here that the behaviour does not have to result in any sort of offence but, rather, it *mirrors* behaviour which was present at the time of an offence.

There has been nothing written specifically on OPB in those with a history of firesetting, which, I argue is an important omission. Below, is a list of considerations which professionals should be aware of when monitoring people who light fires. Much of this information will likely be gleaned from observational data over a period of time, and this emphasises the importance of clinical record keeping. Important considerations should include:

- Is there anything of note about the service user's interactions with non-flame sources of heat, such as hot water? For example, they might engage in self-harm through the use of boiling water;
- Does the service user make any particular references to fire in conversation?
- Do they make any verbal threats involving references to fire, e.g. 'I will torch you' or 'I will burn your house down'?
- Do they show particular interest in news stories involving fire/arson? For example, in assessing those who set fires, I routinely enquire about their response to the news about the Grenfell tower block fire in June 2017;
- Is there evidence of any physiological arousal to fire-related stimuli?
- Is there any evidence of institutional firesetting (i.e. in prison or hospital)?
- If the service user does have any opportunity to interact with fire directly, for instance in cookery classes, how do they behave?
- What is the service user's response if they are in the presence of the fire brigade/fire alarms?
- Be aware of the individual's presentation on and around celebrations which involve fire, for example, 'bonfire night' in November and religious festivals such as Diwali;
- Be aware of very subtle parallels to fire in the service user's behaviour and presentation. For example, if they attend art classes, do they tend to select particular colours associated with fire such as red or yellow? This should be explored with them.

Summary

In this chapter I have proposed that adopting a holistic perspective on fire *use* could enhance the assessment of those who light fires by forensic psychologists and allied professionals. The suggestions in this chapter are designed to aid practitioners in tailoring the assessment process; moving away from the 'one size fits all' approach which has traditionally been adopted. The utility of the dimensional conceptualisation of fire use has been highlighted. We should consider a service user's history with fire, which is potentially an important predisposing factor. There are also important dynamic predisposers to be considered, in addition to the need for a thorough offence account and collecting information on what might have precipitated it. Throughout this chapter, an emphasis has been placed on understanding the importance of cultural background; this is not, in my opinion, stressed enough in our work with those who light fires currently and is a research priority. Lastly, in monitoring risk, I have suggested two areas worthy of consideration, namely self-preservation strategies (which should inform treatment planning – see Chapter 7) and offence paralleling behaviour. High quality forensic risk assessments should be holistic and collaborative and should be used to identify an individual's needs. These needs can be addressed in treatment, which is discussed in the next chapter.

Treatment and intervention with people who set fires

7

Overview

Until relatively recently, options for the rehabilitative treatment of those convicted of firesetting offences were limited. In the prison service in England and Wales the 'one size fits all' approach already discussed in relation to assessment in the previous chapter, also applied to treatment. In practice, this meant that convicted people would typically participate in generic treatment programmes rather than having access to an approach specifically tailored to their needs.

The recently developed the firesetter intervention programme for prisoners (FIPP, Gannon, 2013; as cited in Gannon et al., 2015) and a version for mentally disordered offenders (FIP-MO; Gannon & Lockerbie, 2011, 2012, 2014; as cited in Tyler et al., 2018) provides a manualised and evidence-based approach to reducing risk in those who light fires. The programmes mark a significant turning point and reflect a new way of thinking, namely that the needs of a person who sets fires may be very different from those of other forensic service users. The FIPP and FIP-MO are still relatively new but early evidence is promising with respect to efficacy (for example see Tyler et al., 2018). There are also other treatments available for those in specialist services, such as the Northgate firesetters treatment programme (Taylor, Thorne, Robertson & Avery, 2002; Taylor, Thorne & Slavkin, 2004; Taylor, Robertson, Thorne, Belshaw & Watson, 2006), which has been running in a forensic learning disability service for over ten years; research indicates post-treatment improvements on psycho-social functioning (Taylor, Thorne & Slavkin, 2004).

The availability of treatment specifically designed for adults who have set fires and reside in prison and hospital settings is important in tackling firesetting.

DOI: 10.4324/9780367808648-7

However, this is a post-offence approach meaning that service users will usually have already set dangerous and reckless fires even before being eligible for treatment. I argue that, alongside rehabilitative treatment, we need to be seeking a holistic and, indeed, sociological solution which takes account of how fire is socially constructed. This relies upon early intervention. More specifically, I suggest that we should be supporting young people to form a healthy relationship with fire from an early age which could, potentially, prevent them from ever engaging in criminalised forms of fire use. This requires a change in messaging surrounding fire, which can best be achieved not only through structured intervention but also on a wider societal level.

In this chapter, the treatment and intervention implications of the continuum of fire use (CoFU) conceptualisation and, specifically, the continuum of fire use theory (CoFUT) are considered, In discussing 'treatment', I am referring to structured programmes targeted at the rehabilitation of adults convicted of firesetting offences. The term 'intervention programmes' relates to structured programmes delivered to young people who are setting fires or thought to be at risk of doing so. Lastly, I use the terms 'intervention' and 'early intervention' in a broader sense to describe any sort of change in thinking and approach which could be applied at a societal level with a view to contributing to firesetting prevention / reduction.

The CoFU

To summarise, a central tenet of this book is that arson / firesetting should be reconceptualised, namely by looking at fire *use* as a dimensional construct. Fire use exists along a continuum – the CoFU. I am arguing that we should be viewing fire use more holistically through seeking to understand the full spectrum, ranging from non-criminalised to criminalised. The CoFU can be applied individually, i.e. to understand the course of an individual's fire use across their lifespan but also to a whole population, to understand the variation from person to person. This advances the current way of thinking in forensic psychology which, so far, has focussed solely on one end of the continuum – criminalised fire use in the form of arson / firesetting. The CoFU encourages a much-needed wider perspective on fire use and is consistent with the strengths-based approach, which now increasingly plays a role in practitioners' work with forensic service users, at least theoretically (see Heffernan & Ward, 2017; Ward, 2017 for examples).

The CoFU epitomises the fluid nature of fire use. In my experience as a researcher and practitioner, any assumption that those convicted of firesetting offences have only ever engaged in criminalised fire use is flawed. Rather, many will have a history of experiences which span the entirety of the CoFU.

With respect to the imprisoned participants in my research (Horsley, 2020) *non-criminalised* fire use always preceded criminalised use; in other words, there is evidence that they progressed along the continuum to the point at which they were reprimanded. The non-imprisoned participants in my study clearly did not follow the same trajectory in that their interactions with fire have remained at the lower end of the continuum. We might, therefore, reasonably surmise that there are protective factors at play in their case but what constitutes a protective factor in relation to fire use is yet to be researched.

I argue that healthy fire-interactions should not be neglected by forensic practitioners and researchers just because of an entrenched bias towards risk. Rather, it is important we learn more about how people engage *adaptively* with fire because this could provide a blueprint for future firesetting treatment and intervention. When working therapeutically, we should acknowledge a service user's adaptive fire use and seek to understand its function, as well as addressing their firesetting. Ideally, a person who lights fires should have the opportunity to *learn* how to engage with fire more adaptively again in the future. Theoretically, therefore, an argument could be made that the cessation approach, i.e. preventing any contact with fire, is unhelpful because it prohibits the reinforcement and practical *learning* of appropriate fire-related behaviour. Enforced cessation from fire use also strengthens the idea that fire is taboo (returned to below) and might only put a temporary stop on a service user's proclivity to re-engage with fire in a criminalised manner at some point in the future. In reality, however, preventing a person who lights fires from having contact with fire is necessary in forensic settings from a safety perspective. This point highlights the cyclical conflict between what makes sense theoretically and what is safe and feasible in forensic contexts. Striking the right balance is difficult but in prisons and forensic hospitals the safety of service users and staff has to supersede all else.

As explained previously, the CoFU is a conceptualisation or way of thinking about fire use, whereas the CoFUT is a specific theory based on the findings of my own research (Horsley, 2020). The next section of this chapter will draw on the CoFUT in terms of its potential to inform treatment and intervention.

The CoFUT

The CoFUT comprises three themes – Transient Emotional State, Sense of Self and Psychological Wellbeing – which depict psychological factors of relevance in the human – fire relationship according to the data from my research (Horsley, 2020). The treatment and intervention implications of the CoFUT are discussed below. First, the relevance of each individual theme is outlined and then wider points are considered, alongside existing literature.

Transient Emotional State

This CoFUT theme is concerned with the immediate positive impact of fire use on emotional state, which is reinforcing, thus increasing the likelihood of future interactions with fire. The finding that fire use has a positive effect on one's emotional state suggests that emotion regulation could be a worthwhile treatment target for those who lights fires. Furthermore, for some of the imprisoned participants in my study (Horsley, 2020) criminalised forms of fire use has provided a route through which to solve interpersonal problems. This suggests there might also be value in addressing interpersonal problem solving in rehabilitative treatment. Encouragingly, emotional regulation and problem solving both feature in existing treatment programmes, such as the FIPP (Gannon, 2013; as cited in Gannon et al., 2015) and FIP-MO (Gannon & Lockerbie, 2011, 2012, 2014; as cited in Tyler et al., 2018) as well as the Northgate firesetters treatment programme (Taylor, Thorne, Robertson & Avery, 2002; Taylor, Thorne & Slavkin, 2004; Taylor, Robertson, Thorne, Belshaw & Watson, 2006).

Although emotion management and problem solving may be worthwhile treatment targets, data supporting the CoFUT Transient Emotional State theme emphasises that the lure of fire's immediately gratifying qualities is very strong. This poses a therapeutic problem. Furthermore, not only is fire attractive on a sensory basis but, for some, the risk associated with criminalised fire use might also be part of its appeal. This is compellingly reminiscent of the sociological concept of edgework (Lyng, 1990, 2005), which is concerned with taking risks and, specifically, the stimulation associated with pushing the boundary between control and chaos. Any form of fire use arguably carries some degree of risk because of fire's potential to damage and harm but the appraisal of this risk is subjective. The notion of control over fire (or, at least, perceived control) was alluded to by many of my participants, as discussed in Chapter 5. Additionally, skill, which is another characteristic of edgework, is of relevance in considering fire use. Fire is inherently dangerous and, thus, interacting with it requires skill. Arguably, anyone who succeeds in at least partly manipulating fire to behave in the way they intend is skilful, even if that manipulation happens to come in the form of an offence. This concept has been discussed in the empirical literature by Butler and Gannon (2015, 2020) who argue that those who set fires have a particular expertise in misusing fire, along with offence-supportive scripts.

Interpreted through the lens of edgework, interacting with fire provides an exhilarating opportunity to push the boundaries, which is likely part of its appeal for those who already have a proclivity towards risk taking. Therefore, if we wish to 'rehabilitate' adults who have set fires, there surely needs to be alternative routes through which they can find the same exhilaration. Replacing a maladaptive goal-orientated behaviour with a more adaptive alternative is the premise of the Good Lives Model (GLM; Ward & Brown, 2004) and is a feature of the FIPP (Gannon, 2013; as cited in Gannon et al., 2015) and FIP-MO (Gannon & Lockerbie, 2011, 2012, 2014; as cited in Tyler et al., 2018) programmes.

I am suggesting here that the appeal of fire use as a form of risk taking must, specifically, be taken in to consideration in the delivery of firesetting treatment. The significance of this is even greater if we accept that there is some connection between the immediately gratifying appeal of fire and the evolution of our species as previously discussed. If we are 'programmed' to find this aspect of fire use attractive then lessening its appeal poses a significant challenge. The challenge, I argue, is particularly great for those practitioners who work with adults convicted of firesetting offences whose behaviour may have become very entrenched over a long period of time through reinforcement - a mechanism referred to in theoretical work by Jackson et al. (1987) and Gannon et al. (2012). On this basis, I suggest that we need to be realistic about how much can be achieved through adult rehabilitative treatment which is delivered *post*-offence.

Above, I have proposed that the extent of the sensory appeal of fire presents a quandary for practitioners and so how could this be resolved? There is an argument that it could be addressed through a process of gradual desensitisation to fire through an approach called *exposure therapy (ET)*. This is already a core component of cognitive behavioural therapy for anxiety and phobia (Craske, Treanor, Conway, Zbozinek & Vervliet, 2014; Weisman & Rodebaugh, 2018). ET comes in many forms, including *gradually* exposing a client to a particular stimulus, *imaginal* exposure to the stimulus or "intense" exposure, which is sometimes referred to as "flooding" (Craske et al., 2014, p. 10). There is an argument, therefore, that this principle could be applied to the treatment of those who set fires. More specifically, repeated exposure to fire in mundane contexts (see below for more discussion) might lead to reduced arousal over time and, thus, could lessen its immediate appeal. In other words, the service user becomes acclimatised to fire and so it is no longer so exciting or memorising.

Exposure to fire may, theoretically, be a useful pursuit in the treatment of those who set fires but the possible benefits are surpassed by safety constraints. Gradually exposing service users who are convicted of firesetting to *actual* fire carries serious risk implications, particularly against the backdrop of other psychological characteristics which are prominent in people who have committed crime such as impulsivity, emotional dysregulation and mental disorder and where individuals are housed in a secure forensic setting. This is another example of the conflict between what may make theoretical sense from a rehabilitative perspective versus what is realistic within the constraints of secure settings like prisons and forensic hospitals. Although the risks associated with intensive ET render it unsafe and, ultimately, infeasible in forensic settings, there are practical alternatives. For example, the FIPP employs "covert satiation" (Gannon et al., 2015, p. 43), which does not require exposure to *actual* fire. Here, service users are asked to imagine scenarios in which they would be tempted to set a fire along with imagining the negative consequences of doing so, for instance, being burnt or seeing a family member cry when they are sentenced in the court room. The idea is that through pairing the firesetting and consequences imagery, the temptation to set fires will weaken over time (T.A. Gannon, personal communication, February 5, 2021).

In the section above, treatment and intervention considerations relating to the Transient Emotional State CoFUT theme were outlined. Next, the second CoFUT theme – Sense of Self – is discussed.

Sense of Self

The Sense of Self strand of the CoFUT exemplifies how fire use impacts on one's identity and self-esteem, which has implications for the treatment of people who set fires. Self-esteem has attracted the attention of arson/firesetting researchers (for example, Day, 2001; Duggan & Shine, 2001; Gannon et al., 2013) and low self-esteem is a feature of theoretical work (for example, Jackson et al., 1987; Gannon et al., 2013). Furthermore, it is addressed directly in the FIPP and FIP-MO, through repeatedly encouraging group members to generate positive self-statements (T.A. Gannon, personal communication, February 5, 2021).

The existing literature suggests that those who light fires might *lack* self-esteem. However, within the CoFUT, a 'boost' to self-esteem can arise from a subjective sense of success in lighting, maintaining and/or interacting with fire. Interestingly, findings from my own research (Horsley, 2020) illuminate possible mediating factors in the connection between fire use and self-esteem, such as peer influence, status and pride, which warrant further exploration through research. From a treatment perspective, it could be helpful to address each of these separately because whereas peer influence might be particularly important for one service user, personal pride might be more relevant for another. Identity, another part of Sense of Self in the CoFUT, does not feature widely in the firesetting literature. However, the fact that Ó Ciardha et al. (2015b) found that identification with fire could distinguish between firesetters and non-firesetters highlights its potential importance. Accordingly, identification with fire is addressed in the FIPP and FIP-MO (T.A. Gannon, personal communication, February 5, 2021).

If we accept that fire can form an important part of users' identity, as represented in the CoFUT, then it follows that these people should be encouraged to strengthen other aspects of their identity to over-ride the importance of fire in their life. This, however, almost certainly sounds more straight forward than it is in practice. I argue that part of the reason why fire plays a role in users' identity is because of the lifelong relationship they have formed with it. Once again, this highlights the potential contribution of early intervention. If young people can be supported in developing a healthy relationship with fire it is more likely to become an adaptive element of their identity. Moreover, if a young person receives the right messaging about fire (see below), it might not even come to form part of their identity at all. That being said, we need to remember that part of our connection with fire is likely innate owing to its role in the evolution of our species which further complicates the role it might play in our identity.

Overall, the Sense of Self CoFUT theme supports the importance of addressing self-esteem and identity in rehabilitative interventions with those who set fires. There might even be value in delving into these concepts further in treatment perhaps, for example, by breaking down self-esteem to explore concepts such as pride. However, I suggest that early intervention offers the most potential in addressing the merging of Sense of Self and fire use. If we can encourage adaptive relationships with fire from an early age, this is surely easier than trying to correct maladaptive relationships which adults have already formed with fire.

The Sense of Self theme feeds into the final CoFUT theme, Psychological Wellbeing, which we will now turn to in relation to forensic treatment and intervention.

Psychological Wellbeing

This CoFUT theme relates to the long-term impact of fire on a user's psychological health. For non-criminalised forms of fire use this appears to be largely positive but for criminalised forms, namely those resulting in sanctions, the effects are negative. In discussing the Psychological Wellbeing theme, I make no claims about the direction of its relationship with fire. In reality, this might be bi-directional or cyclical. In other words, just as fire use impacts on psychological wellbeing, the state of one's psychological wellbeing might also help to determine how they engage with fire. Notwithstanding this, from the narratives of participants in my study (Horsley, 2020) it seems that fire use certainly interacts with psychological health in some way and it is this which forms the basis of the discussion below.

Non-criminalised forms of fire use, culminate in a sense of emotional security (one of the CoFUT sub-themes), which contributes to overall psychological wellbeing. It is possible that this sense of security serves a protective function, meaning that the user is deterred from seeking out more risky or maladaptive forms of fire use and so they remain at the lower end of the continuum. Within the CoFUT the Security sub-theme represents positive qualities of fire such as authenticity, reassurance, positivity, optimism and hope. If, therefore, this is what can be achieved through adaptive interactions with fire, then perhaps emotional security could be a worthwhile treatment target for those convicted of firesetting offences, using the Good Lives Model (GLM; Ward & Brown, 2004) as a framework. More specifically, people who light fires should be supported in identifying pro-social routes through which to achieve a sense of authenticity, reassurance and so on in their lives, such as through art therapy (Gussak, 2009) or meditation, which has been found to have psychological benefits for those with a criminal history (Hawkins, 2003). Broadly, these concepts already feature in the GLM (Ward & Brown, 2004) in the form of primary human goods such as inner peace and spirituality (p. 249). However, how able service users are to truly achieve a sense of security and peace while in prison or a forensic hospital is debatable and so perhaps these should be longer-term goals.

From a treatment perspective, whilst it is important to understand how non-criminalised forms of fire use *enhance* psychological wellbeing through engendering emotional security, we also need to know how criminalised forms of fire use *erode* it. More specifically, the imprisoned participants in my research (Horsley, 2020) speak of the psychologically harmful effects of being stigmatised as an arsonist or firesetter, which leads them to employ self-preservation strategies in order to cope. The way in which we conceptualise these coping strategies determines whether or not they are considered a necessary treatment target for those who light fires. Historically, the externalisation of blame and/or excuse making by those who have committed crime was denounced and deemed to be a negative risk indicator, particularly in the field of sexual offending where the majority of research has been conducted. Consequently, sex-offender treatment programmes included components where service users were encouraged to develop more objective accounts of their offending with a view to correcting their 'distorted thinking' (Auburn & Lea, 2003, p. 281). However, Maruna and Mann (2006) argue such cognitions are equally common in non-forensic populations and should not necessarily be pathologised. Indeed, at some point in our lives we have likely all made excuses or minimised our actions in order to present ourselves more favourably.

With this in mind, and in the spirit of the strengths-based approach, although the self-preservation strategies being employed by those who light fires might be socially undesirable, they may actually be serving a protective function for the individual. Therefore, such strategies should not necessarily be challenged in treatment and, instead, we should be seeking to bolster psychological wellbeing in other ways and, also, to strengthen self-esteem and non-fire-related identity as discussed above. In turn, this tactic could mitigate the psychological threat posed by the arsonist/firesetter 'label'. That being said, there are times where cognitions (such as those I have described as self-preservation strategies) do need to be addressed if they are actually impeding a service user's progress. For example, if a person in prison does not believe that their fire use is problematic, this could mean that they refuse to engage in treatment like the FIPP or FIP-MO. In these cases, it makes sense to support the service user in developing more helpful cognitions and this is best achieved through adopting a compassionate style and with the strengths-based approach in mind.

So far in this chapter, practical applications of the CoFUT in terms of treatment and early intervention have been discussed. In my view, the latter holds the most promise on the premise that it is easier to shape a young person's relationship with fire than it is to 're-write' an adult's (particularly if that adult's behaviour has been continually reinforced). All of this is closely intertwined with cultural considerations, including how fire is socially constructed. The discussion below will focus, specifically, on the potential benefits of early intervention, from a sociological and cultural perspective.

Early intervention

Culture and fire use

As discussed previously, in western culture we are most familiar with fire as a form of entertainment (Fessler, 2006; Winder, 2009) and with the symbolism attached to it (Winder, 2009). There is, I argue, an air of mystery, magic and intrigue surrounding fire. In the UK, we are less often reminded of the functional significance of fire, i.e. our reliance on it for survival. Conversely, in some countries in the Global South (including the community studied by Fessler, 2006), fire in its rawest form – the naked flame – still plays a central role in daily life.

I suggest that in the UK we could learn from the way in which fire is utilised functionally in other countries and cultures and how this impacts on the way it is socially constructed. This knowledge could feed in to how we approach firesetting reduction and prevention. For example, it could be argued that for those using fire very regularly as a functional tool, its impact on individuals' senses and overall emotional state might be less pronounced; a point which is supported by Fessler (2006) and referred to by Ó Ciardha and Gannon (2012). In other words, it is possible that people living in countries and specific communities where fire is used functionally have become sensitised to its stimulating and alluring properties – a concept referred to as habituation (Murray et al., 2015). Likewise, in cultures where fire holds less symbolic and spiritual significance then, perhaps, it would have less relevance to a person's Sense of Self.

In presenting this perspective, i.e. that more functional exposure leads to less interest in it, it is important to highlight a conflicting viewpoint. There has been decades of psychological research on the *mere exposure effect*, which is the idea that individuals tend to show preference to stimuli that they are exposed to repeatedly (Zajonc, 1968). This would suggest, therefore, that the more children are exposed to fire, the more they come to like it. Indeed, this has support from Murray et al. (2015) who found that higher self-reported frequency of fire-exposure in childhood related to higher positivity toward fire in adulthood and a higher likelihood of having used fire for entertainment purposes. This research, therefore, would suggest that actually the more a person is exposed to fire, the more they come to like it. In reality, however, whether repeated exposure to fire leads to liking or habituation is a highly nuanced matter. For example, Murray et al., suggest this might depend on the *frequency* of exposure and Sherrell (2021) also refers to the *type* of exposure, which I believe are likely culture-dependent.

The discussion above highlights an important limitation of the CoFUT, namely that it is grounded in the data from my UK-based study and the themes, such as Transient Emotional State, do not necessarily apply cross-culturally. So what are the implications of culture for early intervention? These are outlined below.

A change in messaging

Notwithstanding the conceptual debate about actual exposure to fire outlined above, I am proposing that a change in messaging about fire in the UK could be helpful. If a more balanced narrative could be relayed to young people then this might, potentially, limit fire's appeal. A shift in the fire-narrative may be achieved through a number of routes, one of which is structured early intervention. Youth intervention programmes for those who set fires already exist; however, there is no standardisation in terms of content or the referral process in England (Foster, 2020a). In fact, Foster highlights the dearth of national guidance for Fire and Rescue Services (FRSs) on the delivery of interventions for young people who light fires, with this being limited to one document published by the Chief Fire Officers Association (CFOA) in 2016 (p. 11). Concerningly, Foster's research found that 30% of UK FRSs rated this document as un-useful (p. 81). Foster (2020a) discusses two forms of firesetting interventions currently offered to young people in the UK, namely fire education programmes which are delivered by FRSs nationwide and psycho-social interventions usually facilitated by clinicians (p. 3). In her research, Foster found that the vast majority of FRSs in the UK offer solely fire safety education (47 out of a total of 53 FRSs surveyed), whereas only four offer a combination of education and psychosocial interventions, with two offering nothing at all. Crucially, existing intervention programmes tend to be targeted; meaning they are aimed at children who are already firesetting or, at least, those who are thought to be at risk of doing so.

In my opinion, the overwhelming emphasis being placed on fire safety means that young people who light fires are almost solely exposed to messages such as 'fire is dangerous' and 'stay away from fire', which may be reinforcing the idea that interacting with fire is taboo. Crucially, primarily educating children only about the *dangers* of fire might, in some cases, be serving to reinforce the intrigue and mystery surrounding it. As outlined in Chapter 6, literature supports the idea that the more forbidden a behaviour, the more compelled young people may be to engage with it; this is referred to by Gannon et al. (2012; p. 19). To recap, Fisher and Birch (1999) offer support for this in the field of child nutrition. They found that when parents restrict access to palatable foods, this can actually encourage the child to seek out the food. In other words, restricting food items "paradoxically may actually promote the very behavior its use is intended to reduce" (p. 1271); I argue that the same stands true for the type of messages we convey about fire.

It is also worth re-emphasising that interventions delivered by FRSs and clinicians are targeted. Whilst there is sense in taking this approach, I also argue that society, more broadly, has a role to play in changing the fire-narrative in the UK. More specifically, not only could fire safety education programmes be increasing the taboo nature of fire use, there is also a risk of children being over-exposed to the exciting, intriguing and glamorous side of fire through the type of messages they receive from a myriad of sources. This point is emphasised by Pinsonneault (2002b, p. 28) who highlights that even the everyday use of fire-related vernacular, such as "carrying a torch" for someone to whom we are attracted might be sending worrisome signals to young children (p. 28).

Interestingly, the school curriculum in England might also be compounding the problem. The key stage one curriculum stipulates that children should be taught about significant events, such as the Great Fire of London (Department of Education, 2013). Online resources offering guidance on how to deliver this material include suggestions of interactive computer games where children can assist fictional characters in extinguishing fires and inviting fire and rescue service personnel to the school in order to demonstrate the extinguishing of a real-fire outdoors (Key Stage History, n.d.). These methods, arguably, run the risk of glamorising fire, thereby increasing the possibility that some children (perhaps those already predisposed to impulsive behaviour and risk-taking) could come to associate it with excitement, intrigue and play. I am not suggesting here that young people should not be learning about such historic and catastrophic events but, perhaps, the mode of delivery and the learning outcomes could benefit from some re-shaping in certain instances. Furthermore, I argue that messages conveying the more mundane side of fire should also be conveyed to children – some examples of the type of messages which might be helpful and how they could be imparted are included in Table 7.1.

Table 7.1 Fire messaging

Message	Questions Suggested teaching topics
Fire and geology	How fire shaped the planet The first occurrences of natural fire, i.e. lightening How the prevalence and form of fire changed over millions of years (drawing on the work of Pyne, 2019)
Fire and evolution	How humans first came to discover fire; the stages of human fire use (i.e. from the first discovery to learning to manipulate it) How fire assisted our ancestors with hunting, gathering and cooking Fire's role in the evolution of our species, such as Wrangham's (2010) work on the cooking hypothesis
Contemporary fire use	The role of fire in the industrial revolution How particular cultures and communities use fire around the world, such as indigenous peoples and populations in the Global South Fire's role in agriculture Fire's 'invisible' role in the UK, such as the workings of gas central heating and gas cookers
The 'down-sides' of fire in the form of the naked flame but *not* with a focus on its dangers	The unpleasantness of smoke, soot and ash The burning of fossil fuels and the impact of this on the environment – this might include discussion on the 'cleaner' alternatives such as wind energy and why this is important

Mundane fire messaging would enable children to learn about the functionality of fire, rather than only being exposed to its powerful, destructive and dangerous nature. It would be helpful if these messages were reinforced through formal education but that would require policy change, which, must have the support of empirical evidence. As already discussed, however, formal education is not necessarily the only route through which young people can learn about the 'other side' of fire. These messages can be conveyed in many ways, including at home by parents and care givers. All of the topics I am suggesting above can, of course, be approached flexibly in line with the young person's stage of development, learning capacity and personal circumstances.

Ultimately, I am suggesting that making fire less of a taboo in our society, and educating young people about its historical and evolutionary significance, as well as its practical utility could help to reframe it as something which is commonplace, mundane and unappealing. In other words, we need to make fire 'boring'. This could support the development of healthier relationships with fire. Furthermore, in terms of targeted intervention, the psycho-social approach should be more widely available, such as that offered by Foster (2020b). This is a more holistic option, rather than only focussing on fire safety. On a societal level, it is unrealistic to expect a de-construction of everything we have ever believed about fire. However, it is possible that we could strive to convey a more balanced message about fire; care-givers, educators and clinicians are central to this.

Having argued for a change in fire messaging, there are some important caveats. Firstly, it is, of course imperative to strike the right balance. I am not suggesting that educating young people about fire safety, the dangers of fire and the consequences of firesetting is not important. On the contrary, it is imperative that children know how to respond in a fire emergency and how to keep themselves safe. Rather, I am arguing for a more *balanced* approach. Young people should learn about the dangers, how to behave safely around fire and what to do in an emergency, but they should also be exposed to the mundane side of fire in order to help to shape the relationship they go on to form with it. Secondly, I am not proposing that this is a failsafe firesetting-prevention strategy. As discussed throughout this book, the complexity of our relationship with fire as a species, combined with its multi-layered social and symbolic meaning, are very significant hurdles. The points I am making could be adopted as part of a package of tools and techniques and could augment existing interventions. Furthermore, there might be particular points in a young person's development where some of the more nuanced messages about fire are most impactful. Indeed, in her work with young people who set fires, Foster (2020b) astutely aligns the key "fire safety messages" with each developmental stage (p. 43). Lastly, it is important to underline that in using the term 'intervention', I am referring to this to include not only structured programmes but also more broadly to encompass the messages children receive from care-givers, teachers and society as a whole.

Another important caveat is the need for more research. In order to inform any change in message, cross-cultural research is required through which we can study how different populations view fire and how this impacts on the way in which they engage with it. If, for example, certain societies are less attracted to fire from a magic, mystery and intrigue perspective, we may be able to learn something from them and this could be integrated into early intervention. On a more nuanced level, of course, we can also learn from individuals who engage with fire adaptively, such as some of the participants in my study (Horsley, 2020).

Summary

In this chapter, I have outlined considerations for the treatment of adults who set fires, underpinned by the CoFUT. Encouragingly, overall, the CoFUT endorses topics which already feature in existing treatment like the FIPP and FIP-MO, such as the focus on covert sensitisation and self-esteem. There is certainly a place for rehabilitative treatment and the early signs are that specialist programmes like the FIPP and FIP-MO offer a great deal of promise. However, in my view, early intervention is the key to firesetting reduction. By this, I am not only referring to structured intervention programmes but also the role of society, more generally, in sending the right messages about fire to young people. Educators, parents, care givers and clinicians have an important role to play. There is, of course, a need to be realistic. Any hope of a complete overhaul in how we think about fire is unlikely. Rather, some subtle changes in how we teach young people about fire, along with high quality targeted inventions such as that designed by Foster (2020b) should be the way forward.

Conclusion   8

Overview

Throughout this book I have advocated for a more holistic approach to under-standing human interactions with fire; and I have made a number of arguments in support of this. The holistic approach should include viewing fire-related behaviour as more than just the act of firesetting. We should consider fire use as a process, comprising a number of stages, which is in contrast to how it has been presented in much of the existing academic literature. The holistic perspective should also involve re-conceptualising fire use as a dimensional construct. In other words, it is fluid and its nature can vary both over a single person's lifespan and also across a population. It is best captured, therefore, on a continuum – the continuum of fire use (CoFU). Additionally, I am advocating for a move away from a uni-disciplinary perspective. When combined with psychology, the dis-ciplines of sociology, criminology, anthropology and even history can offer a great deal of insight into fire use. Lastly, I propose that more of a focus on the social construction of fire is required. This includes consideration of the way in which our species first came to use fire and how this use has evolved over time, as well as its relevance as a form of symbolism and entertainment. Ultimately, I am suggesting that all of this can enhance our understanding of firesetting and arson and inform the work of forensic psychologists and allied professionals.

All of the arguments summarised above and expounded upon throughout this book share one common attribute; that is, they pertain to the human-fire relationship. This relationship is key to making progress in research and clinical work with those who light fires but it has seldom been acknowl-edged in the forensic psychological literature. This is despite the fact that

DOI: 10.4324/9780367808648-8

anthropogenic fire use dates back millions of years, despite the countless forms of symbolism associated with fire, despite the strength of emotion which fire can evoke and despite our ongoing reliance on fire in daily life.

This final chapter seeks to synthesise the aforementioned core arguments, provide a summary of their potential application and consider future directions.

A holistic conceptualisation of fire use

The study of arson and firesetting has been much neglected when compared to other areas within forensic psychology. Research attention has grown in recent years and this has resulted in some important milestones, such as the development of the M-TTAF (Gannon et al., 2012) and the exploration of non-convicted samples of people who light fires (Gannon & Barrowcliffe, 2012; Barrowcliffe & Gannon, 2015, 2016). Notwithstanding contemporary developments, a number of issues remain. So far, existing research and theory has focused overwhelmingly on firesetting which has resulted in imprisonment/ hospitalisation. There has been a preoccupation, therefore, with what could be appraised as pathological, risky and dangerous interactions with fire. I have argued that this is inconsistent with current directions, for example, the increasing influence of positive psychology (Seligman et al., 2005), which endorses a focus on constructive characteristics and behaviour. With this in mind, therefore, it makes sense to consider the many positives of fire use, as well as understanding the negatives.

Grounded in data from my doctoral research (Horsley, 2020) I developed the first theory of fire *use* – the CoFUT, comprising three themes: Transient Emotional State, Sense of Self and, Psychological Wellbeing. The CoFUT represents the psychological factors and mechanisms underpinning fire use. Albeit preliminary, it provides a novel way of thinking about fire use because it accounts for the full spectrum ranging from non-criminalised to criminalised, rather than only focussing on the latter. Importantly, the CoFUT highlights commonalities in the psychology of fire use, irrespective of the nature of that use (i.e. where it might sit upon the continuum), which reinforces the argument for a dimensional conceptualisation. Of significance is that all of the 24 participants in my research reported an *array* of fire-related experiences, which supports the assertion that it is not always possible to neatly categorise a person as a non-criminalised or criminalised fire user. This highlights limitations to the 'non-firesetter versus firesetter' dichotomy which has commonly been employed in empirical research to date (for examples, see Ducat, McEwan & Ogloff, 2013;

Gannon & Barrowcliffe, 2012; Barrowcliffe & Gannon 2015, 2016). For instance, even if a particular research participant does not have any convictions on record and does not report having engaged in the most severe forms of firesetting, this does not necessarily mean that they have never engaged with fire in a way which approaches the criminalised end of the spectrum. Another important finding to emerge from my research is that participants made reference to different aspects of fire use, from which I developed the stage model. The fundamental point here is that the lighting (or setting) of a fire is only one part of our interaction with it and, thus, a more nuanced examination of fire-related behaviour is required, both in terms of future research but also in clinical practice with those who light fires.

Adopting a broader conceptualisation of fire use (rather than solely fire*setting*) is required to better understand the human-fire relationship. Of equal importance is to consider the social construction of fire.

The social construction of fire

The social construction of fire is integral to a holistic understanding of the human-fire relationship. This concept is itself, multi-layered, comprising manifold interrelated factors such as religion, culture, ethnicity, social norms and legislative frameworks to name but a few. I consider cultural background to be of particular relevance in understanding how fire is socially constructed, not least because it, conceivably, encompasses many of the other factors (i.e. religion, ethnicity and social norms). Fessler (2006) and Winder (2009) hint at the cultural diversity of fire use and, importantly, fire-related symbolism. Indeed, we need only note the array of uses of fire across the globe to appreciate the way this varies across different cultures. For example, consider the ritualistic use of fire handling by Holiness snake handlers in Southern Appalachia (Kane, 1982) and the Northern Greek ritual of fire walking (Danforth, 1989).

Understanding the evolutionary role of fire is also of central importance because it has shaped the way we have come to view fire today and, indeed, the way we interact with it (Horsley, 2020). We, therefore, need to have some appreciation of how human engagement with fire has waxed and waned throughout history because this, too, feeds into how it is socially constructed. Despite fire's central role in the evolution of our species (for discussions see Clark & Harris, 1985; Goudsblom, 1992; Pyne, 1998; Wrangham et al., 1999; Fessler, 2006; Wrangham, 2010; Wrangham & Carmody, 2010), it features sparsely in the psychological literature, which supports the argument for a multi-disciplinary approach to this field of study.

Applications

I am arguing that a change in perspective and a change in messaging could be advantageous for the work of forensic practitioners and researchers in understanding and reducing firesetting. The potential application of these ideas is summarised below, with respect to forensic assessment and treatment/intervention.

Assessment

Chapter 6 considered the potential applications of a change in the way we think about fire in terms of forensic assessment. For example, I suggested that Canter and Fritzon's work (1998) could be applied in collecting information on fire use history and that an offence account could be broken down into stages. I also introduced the three polarities, which build on the work of Ó Ciardha et al. (2015b). The three polarities (i.e. taboo - non-taboo; magical/mysterious – mundane, and; functional – non-functional/entertainment), should be investigated through research but they also have clinical utility. The polarities are a useful depiction of the variability in different people's views on fire, which, I argue is likely a function of cultural background amongst other factors. I suggest that the CoFUT also has the potential to enhance the assessment of people who set fires. More specifically, the three themes (Transient Emotional State, Sense of Self and Psychological Wellbeing) should form part of an interview session with a service user in order to explore the role which fire has played in their lives and psyche. The CoFUT can also inform risk monitoring and management, as exemplified by the discussion on risk paralleling behaviours in Chapter 6.

Treatment and intervention

As expounded in Chapter 7, the CoFUT is of relevance in planning treatment for adults who light fires. It offers support for existing programmes, such as the FIPP (Gannon, 2013; as cited in Gannon et al., 2015) and FIP-MO (Gannon & Lockerbie, 2011, 2012, 2014; as cited in Tyler et al., 2018) whilst also illuminating topics which might benefit from further consideration. Crucially, although rehabilitative programmes offer promise, I suggest that early intervention is key, both in terms of targeted intervention programmes and also with respect to the fire messages children receive from society more widely. I have argued in this book that a change in the way we think about fire in the UK could, potentially, reduce its appeal to young people as a source of play, excitement and risk-taking.

Currently, I suggest that fire is portrayed as taboo in the UK and it is possible that this might be serving to increase young people's interest in it. A change of direction could see children having more exposure to the mundane and functional side of fire. If we can shape healthy relationships with fire from an early age and reduce the mystery and intrigue surrounding it then this could, potentially, prove to be a positive preventative strategy. Of course more research is required to explore this idea but, theoretically, it has support from Fessler (2006) who noted a relative absence of risky fire-related behaviour amongst children in a community where they engaged with fire functionally, and very regularly, from a very early age.

The crux of the above argument is that early intervention is key to reducing firesetting. Currently, fire and rescue services (FRSs) in the UK are largely responsible for delivering fire safety education programmes, with the availability of psychosocial interventions being sparse (Foster, 2020a). Ideally, the latter should be more widely available, such as the approach offered by Foster (2020b). However, the wider societal approach I am calling for has an important role to play in a change of message relayed to children and this can be supported by teachers, caregivers and clinicians. Ultimately, if we accept that fire and fire use are social constructs then this means that firesetting is a *social* problem. It cannot and should not be understood as a problem *within* one individual (this is often the focus of mainstream forensic psychology, or, at least traditionally it has been). Rather, it should be understood as a consequence of the way we, as a society, view fire. This highlights the importance of drawing on sociological work. Currently, in my experience, existing treatment and intervention programmes have a heavy psychological focus, which is arguably somewhat insular.

Thinking outside the box

With some creative thinking the ideas being proposed in this book can be applied more widely to improve practice and research in other areas. First and foremost, I am arguing that adopting a multi-disciplinary approach to understanding fire use and tackling firesetting is a helpful way forward. There is, therefore, the potential for closer working between scholars from different disciplines, including practitioners and researchers. One example of this is the potential influence of anthropological work. As discussed in Chapter 2, Sandgathe (2017) refers to the lack of consensus surrounding when our ancestors first started to use fire. There is also a lack of clarity on how, exactly, we first came to use it. Fessler (2006) suggests this may have resulted from early fire play as our ancestors observed sparks arising from their use of flint to fashion tools. There is an emphasis throughout this book, therefore, on the role of fire use in the evolution of our species but is there any evidence of early criminalised use (or, at least, what we might identify as criminalised use today)? In other words, if an ability to control fire is admired and provides one with a sense of power (as indicated by data from my research – Horsley, 2020), then is there any evidence that our ancestors *mis*used it as a means of attracting mates? Evolutionary perspectives on other forms of offending exist. For instance, in the confluence model of sexual aggression, Malamuth (1996, as cited in Ward et al., 2006) proposes that an important factor in male sexual offending against women is males' desire for reproductive success. Therefore, there is scope to explore a similar perspective in relation to arson/ firesetting, albeit there are challenges with archaeological data and it is difficult to distinguish with any certainty between different forms of fire (Sandgathe, 2017).

I suggest that there is potential for anthropology to feed into the design of firesetting treatment. In my experience, the development of structured programmes is often uni-disciplinary. Prison Service-run programmes, for example, tend to have a psycho-social focus. I have direct experience of facilitating and managing a number of these programmes and I have certainly never seen reference to experts from alternative disciplinary backgrounds being extensively consulted. There is vast potential for the consultation of academics and practitioners with an anthropology background and this marks an exciting opportunity for future collaboration.

Sociology is another discipline which should be drawn upon more widely to move research and practice forward. Ultimately, in my view, fire and fire use are at least partly social constructs and, therefore, arson/firesetting is a *social* problem. This highlights the importance of drawing on sociological work in order to understand it and this could also include incorporating historical perspectives. For instance, how have societal views about fire evolved? In Chapter 3, I made reference to the 18th century practice of burning at the stake in England. We could learn more about how to target the contemporary fire message from tracking how it has changed over time. As already discussed, I believe that the change of message which I am arguing for can be best achieved through community-orientated interventions. There are, therefore, opportunities for closer collaboration between practitioner psychologists and other professionals, such as social workers, probation officers and youth workers. In my opinion, co-working, specifically in reference to the development of early interventions targeting anti-social behaviour and crime, does not happen enough.

Alongside better multi-disciplinary working, another possible wider application of the ideas being proposed in this book is that they could extend beyond firesetting. I suggest that at least some of the key arguments I have made can apply to other behaviours, such as risky sexual practices, drug-taking and dangerous driving. For example, in writing about risky leisure Berdychevsky (2018) explains that despite usually being socially constructed as 'deviant', sadomasochistic activities and BDSM (Bondage and Discipline, Sadism and Masochism) have been found to offer psychological benefits for those who *consensually* engage in it (Franklin-Reible, 2006, as cited in Berdychevsky, 2018, p. 13). This example hints at the many opportunities for opening up the way we think about criminalised, taboo and/or socially demonised behaviours as being dimensional and nuanced rather than simply 'right' or 'wrong'. Ultimately, adopting a more holistic view could help to encourage adaptive behaviour and, indeed, aid the recognition of unsafe behaviour from a public health perspective.

Similarly, it is easy to see how the tenet about *pre-emptively* seeking to help young people develop a healthy relationship with fire could apply elsewhere, such as with sexual behaviour, illicit substances, gambling and so on. I am not suggesting that these are new ideas; indeed, the field of cultural criminology (Hayward, 2015, as cited in Smith & Raymen, 2018) already has much to offer. However, I am seeking to highlight that the way of thinking which I am promoting with respect to firesetting could be applied more widely. It can complement existing research and practice, as well as promoting a new look at topics which have traditionally been taboo and/or reduced to the deviant/non-deviant or illegal/legal dichotomy.

Future directions

An interdisciplinary approach, drawing on anthropology, sociology, criminology and even history, could enhance clinical practice with people who light fires but this must, of course, be predicated on good research. There are, in my view, a number of priorities for future research. The social construction of fire use is an important topic. This should include studies into the role that cultural background plays in the way a person views fire and, consequently, how they use it. Findings from this research could inform approaches to the assessment of people with a firesetting history and, crucially, treatment and intervention strategies. In the future, the Fire Use Matrix (FUM) could be used as a research tool but first it requires refinement. There are also other areas which require more work. For example, fire interest and fire-supportive attitudes are potentially extremely important factors in understanding fire use but research is in its relative infancy (see Ó Ciardha et al., 2015a,b). Also, the role of early exposure to fire, building on the work of Murray et al., (2015) and Sherrell (2021), is a promising avenue for further study. Additionally, there is a need for more qualitative research exploring fire use. In particular, the notion that fire is a taboo topic in the UK and how this could, potentially, increase intrigue and excitement in young people requires exploration. More specifically, a qualitative exploration of the types of messages which are relayed to children about fire (i.e. 'fire is forbidden') would be helpful. This could inform early interventions aiming to change the message to one which promotes healthy interactions and, thus, relationships with fire. Broadly speaking, I argue that future research should adopt a dimensional perspective on fire use; rather than seeking to draw dichotomies like 'firesetter/ non-firesetter'.

Summary

The arguments made within this book are based not only on research findings but also on my 15 years of experience as a practitioner forensic psychologist, through which I have worked with people who light fires. I have argued for a re-conceptualisation of fire use from categorical to dimensional. I have developed a new, albeit preliminary, theory – the CoFUT – which is grounded in data from my doctoral research. Furthermore, I have argued that we should consider fire use as a process, rather than a single event. I have suggested that psychology cannot address all that we need to learn about fire use as a standalone discipline and, thus, an interdisciplinary approach is required. In my view, we are only ever going to have an impoverished and limited understanding of arson/ firesetting unless we broaden our perspective. We must better understand non-criminalised fire use and we must better acknowledge historical, evolutionary and sociological perspectives. I argue that without adopting a more holistic conceptualisation we are limited in what can be achieved in the firesetting field. The ideas presented within this book promote a change in direction in forensic psychology but I am also advocating for a change in the way that we, as a society, think about fire. This type of shift will take time and, ultimately, more research is required to support it. If progress is to be made in the future, there may also need to be policy change; however, again, this will only come about through more research.

Humans share a very long and complex relationship with fire and its symbolic significance is very powerful. Ultimately, in order to interact safely with fire, people need to have a healthy relationship with it. The shaping of this relationship needs to start early in life. We must dedicate time and resources to early intervention strategies for young people. After all, when writing a story, it is surely easier to get it right the first time than to have to erase it and start all over again.

References

Andrews, D. A., & Bonta, J. (2014). *The Psychology of Criminal Conduct*. Oxon, England: Routledge.

Antonowicz, D. H., & Ross, R. R. (2005). Social problem-solving deficits in offenders. *Social Problem Solving and Offending: Evidence, Evaluation and Evolution* (pp. 91–102). Chichester: Wiley.

Auburn, T., & Lea, S. (2003). Doing cognitive distortions: A discursive psychology analysis of sex offender treatment talk. *British Journal of Social Psychology, 42*(2), 281–298. doi: 10.1348/014466603322127256

Averill, S. (2010). Legal perspectives on arson. In G. L. Dickens, P. A. Sugarman & T. A. Gannon (Eds.). *Firesetting and Mental Health* (pp. 165–184). London, England: RCPsych Publications.

Barnoux, M., Gannon, T. A., & Ó Ciardha, C. (2015). A descriptive model of the offence chain for imprisoned adult male firesetters (descriptive model of adult male firesetting). *Legal and Criminological Psychology, 20*(1), 48–67.

Barrowcliffe, E. R., & Gannon, T. A. (2015). The characteristics of un-apprehended firesetters living in the UK community. *Psychology, Crime & Law, 21*(9), 836–853. doi: 10.1080/1068316X.2015.1054385

Barrowcliffe, E. R., & Gannon, T. A. (2016). Comparing the psychological characteristics of un-apprehended firesetters and non-firesetters living in the UK. *Psychology, Crime & Law, 22*(4), 382–404. doi: 10.1080/1068316X.2015.1111365

Barrowcliffe, E. R., Gannon, T. A., & Tyler, N. (2019). Measuring the cognition of firesetting individuals using explicit and implicit measures. *Psychiatry, 82*(4), 368–371.

BBC (2009). Hanukkah. Retrieved from: https://www.bbc.co.uk/religion/religions/judaism/holydays/hanukkah.shtml

Bell, R. (2016). Working with adult arsonists. In R. M. Doley, G. L. Dickens & G. A. Gannon (Eds.). *The Psychology of Arson* (pp. 41–54). Oxon, England: Routledge.

Berdychevsky, L. (2018). "Risky" leisure research on sex and violence: Innovation, impact, and impediments. *Leisure Sciences, 40*(1–2), 9–18.

Blumenthal, S., Gudjonsson, G., & Burns, J. (1999). Cognitive distortions and blame attribution in sex offenders against adults and children. *Child Abuse & Neglect, 23*(2), 129–143. doi: 10.1016/S0145-2134(98)00117-3

Botoeva, G. (2019). Use of language in blurring the lines between legal and illegal. In A. Polese, A. Russo & F. Strazzari (Eds.). *Governance beyond the Law: The Illegal, the Immoral and the Criminal* (pp. 67–83). Cham, Switzerland: Palgrave Macmillan.

Braun, V., & Clarke, V. (2013). *Successful Qualitative Research: A Practice Guide for Beginners.* London: Sage.

Brett, A. (2004). Kindling theory' in arson: How dangerous are firesetters? *Australian and New Zealand Journal of Psychiatry*, 38(6), 419–425. doi: 10.1080/j.1440-1614.2004.01378.x

Britt, M. E. (2011). *Playing with Fire or Arson? Identifying Predictors of Juvenile Firesetting Behavior* (unpublished masters dissertation). University of Nevada, Las Vegas, United State of America. Retrieved from: https://digitalscholarship.unlv.edu/cgi/viewcontent.cgi?referer=https://scholar.google.co.uk/&httpsredir=1&article=1984&context=thesesdissertations

Brown, J., Shell, Y., & Cole, T. (2015). *Forensic Psychology: Theory, Research, Policy and Practice.* London: Sage.

Burke, P. J., & Stets, J. E. (2009). *Identity Theory.* Oxon, England: Oxford University Press.

Butler, H., & Gannon, T. A. (2015). The scripts and expertise of firesetters: A preliminary conceptualization. *Aggression and Violent Behavior*, 20, 72–81. doi:10.1016/j.avb.2014.12.011

Butler, H., & Gannon, T. A. (2020). Do deliberate firesetters hold fire-related scripts and expertise? A quantitative investigation using fire service personnel as comparisons. *Psychology, Crime & Law*, 1–21.

Campbell, R. (1984). Sentence of death by burning for women. *The Journal of Legal History*, 5(1), 44–59. doi: 10.1080/01440368408530794

Canter, D., & Fritzon, K. (1998). Differentiating arsonists: A model of firesetting actions and characteristics. *Legal and Criminological Psychology*, 3(1), 73–96. doi: 10.1111/j.2044-8333.1998.tb00352.x

Charmaz, K. (1990). Discovering chronic illness: Using grounded theory. *E-Journal of Social Science & Medicine*, 30(11), 1161–1172. Retrieved from https://www.journals.elsevier.com/social-science-and-medicine

Clark, J. D., & Harris, J. W. (1985). Fire and its roles in early hominid lifeways. *E-Journal of African Archaeological Review*, 3(1), 3–27. Retrieved from https://link.springer.com/journal/10437

Clipper, W. (2007). Burning Man: Festival culture in the United States – Festival culture in a global perspective. In T. Hauptfleisch, S. Lev-Aladgem, J. Martin, W. Sauter & H. Schoenmakers (Eds.). *Festivalising! Theatrical Events, Politics and Culture* (pp. 221–241). New York, NY: The John Hopkins University Press.

Craske, M. G., Treanor, M., Conway, C. C., Zbozinek, T., & Vervliet, B. (2014). Maximizing exposure therapy: An inhibitory learning approach. *Behaviour Research and Therapy*, 58, 10–23. doi: 10.1016/j.brat.2014.04.006

Dalhuisen, L., Koenraadt, F., & Liem, M. (2015). Psychotic versus non-psychotic firesetters: Similarities and differences in characteristics. *The Journal of Forensic Psychiatry & Psychology*, 26(4), 439–460. doi: 10.1080/14789949.2015.1018927

Dalhuisen, L., Koenraadt, F., & Liem, M. (2017). Subtypes of firesetters. *Criminal Behaviour and Mental Health*, 27(1), 59–75.

Dallos, R., Stedmon, J., & Johnstone, L. (2014). Integrative formulation in theory. In L. Johnstone & R. Dallos (Eds.) *Formulation in Psychology and Psychotherapy*. East Sussex, England: Routledge.

Danforth, L. (1989). *Firewalking and Religious Healing: The Anastenaria of Greece and the American Firewalking Movement.* Princeton, NJ: Princeton University Press. Retrieved from http://www.jstor.org/stable/j.ctt1dxg8pg

Davis, J. A., & Lauber, K. M. (1999). Criminal behavioral assessment of arsonists, pyromaniacs, and multiple firesetters: The burning question. *Contemporary Criminal Justice, 15*(3), 273–290. doi.org/10.1177/1043986299015003005

Day, J. (2001). Understanding the characteristics of fire-setters. *Prison Service Journal,* (133), 6–8.

Daykin, A., & Hamilton, L. (2012). Arson. In Winder, B., & Banyard, P. (Eds.). *A Psychologist's Casebook of Crime: From Arson to Voyeurism.* Hampshire, England: Palgrave Macmillan.

Department of Education (2013). The National Curriculum in England: History Programmes of Study. Retrieved from: https://www.gov.uk/government/publications/national-curriculum-in-england-history-programmes-of-study/national-curriculum-in-england-history-programmes-of-study#key-stage-2.

Dickens, G. L., & Sugarman, P. A. (2012). Adult firesetters: Prevalence, characteristics and psychopathology. In G. Dickens & P. Sugarman (Eds.). *Firesetting and Mental Health* (pp. 3–27). London, England: RC Psych Publications.

Dickens, G., Sugarman, P., Edgar, S., Hofberg, K., Tewari, S., & Ahmad, F. (2009). Recidivism and dangerousness in arsonists. *The Journal of Forensic Psychiatry & Psychology, 20*(5), 621–639. doi: 10.1080/14789940903174006

Dobson, J. L. (2009). Learning style preferences and course performance in an undergraduate physiology class. *Advances in Physiology Education, 33*(4), 308–314

Dolan, M., Millington, J., & Park, I. (2002). Personality and neuropsychological function in violent, sexual and arson offenders. *Medicine, Science and the Law, 42*(1), 34–43. doi: 10.1177/002580240204200107

Doley, R. (2003). Making sense of arson through classification. *E-Journal of Psychiatry, Psychology and Law, 10*(2), 346–352. Retrieved from https://www.tandfonline.com/loi/tppl20

Doley, R. M., Dickens, G. L., & Gannon, T. A. (2016). Introduction: Deliberate firesetting – An overview. In R. M. Doley, G. L. Dickens & T. A. Gannon (Eds.). *The Psychology of Arson: A Practical Guide to Understanding and Managing Deliberate Firesetters* (pp. 1–11). Oxon, England: Routledge.

Douglas, K. S., & Skeem, J. L. (2005). Violence risk assessment: Getting specific about being dynamic. *Psychology, Public Policy, and Law, 11*(3), 347

Ducat, L., McEwan, T., & Ogloff, J. R. (2013). Comparing the characteristics of firesetting and non-firesetting offenders: Are firesetters a special case? *The Journal of Forensic Psychiatry & Psychology, 24*(5), 549–569

Ducat, L., McEwan, T. E., & Ogloff, J. R. (2015). An investigation of firesetting recidivism: Factors related to repeat offending. *Legal and Criminological Psychology, 20*(1), 1–18. doi: 10.1111/lcrp.12052

Dudley, R., & Kuyken, W. (2014). Formulation in cognitive behavioural therapy: A principle driven approach. In L. Johnstone & R. Dallos (Eds.). *Formulation in Psychology and Psychotherapy: Making Sense of People's Problems* (pp. 18–44). Sussex, England: Routledge.

Duggan, L., & Shine, J. (2001). An investigation of the relationship between arson, personality disorder, hostility, neuroticism and self-esteem amongst incarcerated fire-setters. *Prison Service Journal,* (133), 18–21.

Edwards, M. J., & Grace, R. C. (2014). The development of an actuarial model for arson recidivism. *Psychiatry, Psychology and Law, 21*(2), 218–230. doi: 10.1080/13218719.2013.803277

Etikan, I., Musa, S. A., & Alkassim, R. S. (2016). Comparison of convenience sampling and purposive sampling. *American Journal of Theoretical and Applied Statistics, 5*(1), 1–4. doi: 10.11648/j.ajtas.20160501.11

Farrington, D. P., Gaffney, H., & Ttofi, M. M. (2017). Systematic reviews of explanatory risk factors for violence, offending, and delinquency. *Aggression and Violent Behavior, 33*, 24–36.

Faulk, M. (1982). The assessment of dangerousness in arsonists. In J. R. Hamilton & H. Freeman (Eds.). *Dangerousness: Psychiatric Assessment and Management* (pp. 73–76). London, England: Gaskell Books.

Fessler, D. M. (2006). A burning desire: Steps toward an evolutionary psychology of fire learning. *Journal of Cognition and Culture, 6*(3), 429–451. doi: 10.1163/156853706778554986

Fineman, K. R. (1995). A model for the qualitative analysis of child and adult fire deviant behaviour. *E-Journal of American Journal of Forensic Psychology, 13*(1), 31–61. https://www.scimagojr.com/journalsearch.php?q=29469&tip=sid&clean=0

Foster, J. E. (2020a). *An Exploratory Study of How Practitioners in UK Fire and Rescue Services Working with Children and Young People Who Set Fires Identify Clients Requiring Psychosocial Interventions* (unpublished master's dissertation). Cambridge University, Cambridge, United Kingdom.

Foster, J. E. (2020b). *Children and Teenagers Who Set Fires; Why They Do It and How to Help.* London, UK: Jessica Kingsley Publishers.

Fradella, H. F. (2007). Why judges should admit expert testimony on the unreliability of eyewitness identifications. *Federal Courts Law Review, 2*, 2–29.

Freud, A. (2018). *The Ego and the Mechanisms of Defence* (revised edition). New York, NY: Routledge.

Fritzen, K. (2012). Theories on arson: The action systems model. In G. L. Dickens, P. A. Sugarman & T. A. Gannon (Eds.). *Firesetting and Mental Health* (pp. 28–47). London, England: RCPsych Publications.

Fritzon, K., Dolan, M., Doley, R., & McEwan, T. E. (2011). Juvenile fire-setting: A review of treatment programs. *Psychiatry, Psychology and Law, 18*(3), 395–408. doi: 10.1080/13218719.2011.585223

Fritzon, K., & Miller, S. (2016). Female firesetters. In R. M. Doley, G. L. Dickens & G. A. Gannon (Eds.). *The Psychology of Arson* (pp. 41–54). Oxon, England: Routledge.

Fisher, J. O., & Birch, L. L. (1999). Restricting access to palatable foods affects children's behavioural response, food selection, and intake. *The American Journal of Clinical Nutrition, 69*(6), 1264–1272. doi: https://doi.org/10.1093/ajcn/69.6.1264

Gallagher-Duffy, J., MacKay, S., Duffy, J., Sullivan-Thomas, M., & Peterson-Badali, M. (2009). The pictorial fire Stroop: A measure of processing bias for fire-related stimuli. *Journal of abnormal child psychology, 37*(8), 1165.

Gannon, T. A. (2010). Female arsonists: Key features, psychopathologies and treatment needs. *Psychiatry: Interpersonal and Biological Processes, 73*, 173–189. doi: 10.1521/psyc.2010.73.2.173

Gannon, T. A., & Barrowcliffe, E. (2012). Firesetting in The general population: The development and validation of the fire setting and fire proclivity scales. *Legal and Criminological Psychology, 17*(1), 105–122. doi: 10.1348/135532510X523203

Gannon, T. A., Ó Ciardha, C.Ó, Barnoux, M. F., Tyler, N., Mozova, K., & Alleyne, E. K. (2013). Male imprisoned firesetters have different characteristics than other imprisoned offenders and require specialist treatment. *Psychiatry: Interpersonal and Biological Processes, 76*(4), 349–364. doi: 10.1521/psyc.2013.76.4.349

Gannon, T. A., Alleyne, E., Butler, H., Danby, H., Kapoor, A., Lovell, T., … Ó Ciardha, C. (2015). Specialist group therapy for psychological factors associated with firesetting: Evidence of a treatment effect from a non-randomized trial with male prisoners. *Behaviour Research and Therapy, 75*, 42–51. https://doi.org/10.1016/j.brat.2015.07.007.

Gannon, T. A., Ciardha, C. Ó, Doley, R. M., & Alleyne, E. (2012). The multi-trajectory theory of adult firesetting (M-TTAF). *Aggression and Violent Behavior, 17*(2), 107–121. doi: 10.1016/j.avb.2011.08.001

Gannon, T. A., Tyler, N., Barnoux, M. F. L., & Pina, A. (2012). Female arsonists and fireset-ters. In G. L. Dickens, P. A. Sugarman & T. A. Gannon (Eds.). *Firesetting and Mental Health: Theory, Research and Practice* (pp. 126–142). London: RCPsychiatrists.

Gannon, T. A., & Pina, A. (2010). Firesetting: Psychopathology, theory and treatment. *Aggression and Violent Behavior, 15*(3), 224–238. doi: 10.1016/j.avb.2010.01.001

Gawronski, B., LeBel, E. P., & Peters, K. R. (2007). What do implicit measures tell us?: Scruti-nizing the validity of three common assumptions. *Perspectives on Psychological Science, 2*(2), 181–193.

Geller, J. L. (1992). Arson in review: From profit to pathology. *Psychiatric Clinics of North America, 15*(3), 623–645. doi: 10.1016/S0193-953X(18)30228-4

Geller, J. L., Fisher, W. H., & Bertsch, G. (1992). Who repeats? A follow-up study of state hos-pital patients' firesetting behavior. *Psychiatric Quarterly, 63*(2), 143–157

Gilmore, L. (2010).*Theater in a Crowded Fire: Ritual and Spirituality at Burning Man*. Berkley, CA: University of California Press. Retrieved from http://www.jstor.org/stable/10.1525/j.cttlppdct

Gilovich, T., Keltner, D., & Nisbett, R. E. (2010). *Social Psychology*. New York, NY: W.W. Norton & Company, Inc.

Goudsblom, J. (1992). The civilizing process and the domestication of fire. *E-Journal of World History, 3*(1), 1–12. Retrieved from http://www.jstor.org/stable/20078510

Gov.UK (2019) Grenfell Tower Inquiry: Phase 1 Report. Retrieved from: https://assets.grenfelltowerinquiry.org.uk/GTI%20-%20Phase%201%20full%20report%20-%20volume%201.pdf

Gowlett, J. A., & Wrangham, R. W. (2013). Earliest fire in Africa: Towards the convergence of archaeological evidence and the cooking hypothesis. *Azania: Archaeological Research in Africa, 48*(1), 5–30. doi: 10.1080/0067270X.2012.756754

Gowlett, J. A. J. 2016 The discovery of fire by humans: A long and convoluted process. *Philo-sophical Transactions of the Royal Society B, 371*: 20150164. http://dx.doi.org/10.1098/rstb.2015.0164

Greenwald, A. G., Banaji, M. R., Rudman, L. A., Farnham, S. D., Nosek, B. A., & Mellott, D. S. (2002). A unified theory of implicit attitutes, stereotypes, self-esteem, and self-concept. *Psychological Review*, 109, 3–25.

Grolnick, W. S., Cole, R. E., Laurenitis, L., & Schwartzman, P. (1990). Playing with fire: A development assessment of children's fire understanding and experience. *Journal of Clini-cal Child Psychology, 19*(2), 128–135.

Gussak, D. (2009). The effects of art therapy on male and female inmates: Advancing the research base. *The Arts in Psychotherapy, 36*(1), 5–12.

Hagenauw, L. A., Karsten, J., Akkerman-Bouwsema, G. J., de Jager, B. E., & Lancel, M. (2015). Specific risk factors of arsonists in a forensic psychiatric hospital. *International Journal of Offender Therapy and Comparative Criminology, 59*(7), 685–700. doi: 10.1177/0306624X13519744

Hall, J. R. (2000). *Children Playing with Fire. National Fire Protection Association. Fire Analysis and Research Division, 2000*. Retrieved from https://yfires.com/documents/yfires_resource/29.pdf

Hardesty, V. A., & Gayton, W. F. (2002). The problem of children and fire: An historical perspective. In D. J. Kolko (Ed.). *Handbook of Firesetting in Children and Youth* (pp. 1–13). London: Academic Press.

Hart, S., Kropp, P. R., & Laws, D. R.; Klaver, J., Logan, C., & Watt, K. A. (2003). Structured Professional Guidelines for Assessing Risk of Sexual Violence. Vancouver, Canada: The Institute Against Family Violence.

Hawkins, M. A. (2003). Effectiveness of the transcendental meditation program in criminal rehabilitation and substance abuse recovery: A review of the research. *Journal of Offender Rehabilitation, 36*(1–4), 47–65

Heffernan, R., & Ward, T. (2017). A comprehensive theory of dynamic risk and protective factors. *Aggression and Violent Behavior, 37*, 129–141. doi:10.1016/j.avb.2017.10.003

Heyman, J. M. (2013). The study of illegality and legality: Which way forward? *Political and Legal Anthropology Review, 36*(304), 322–326. doi: 10.1111/plar.12030

Higgins, E. T. (1987). Self-discrepancy: A theory relating self and affect. *Psychological Review, 94*(3), 319. doi: 0033-295X/87/S00.75

Home Office (2020). Firs Statistics Data Tables: Deliberate Fires Attended 2020. Retrieved from: https://www.gov.uk/government/statistical-data-sets/fire-statistics-data-tables#deliberate-fires

Hood, J. C. (2007). Orthodoxy vs. Power: The defining traits of grounded Theory. In A. Bryant & K. Charmaz (Eds.). *The Sage Handbook of Grounded Theory* (pp. 151–164). London, England: Sage.

Hope, J. (2018). *Legitimate and Illegitimate Fire-use: A Conceptual Analysis* (unpublished masters dissertation). Newcastle University, Newcastle, England.

Horsley, F. K. (2020). *Arson Reconceptualised: The Continuum of Fire Use* (unpublished doctoral dissertation). Durham University, Durham, United Kingdom.

Horsley, F. K. (2021) Arson and fire setting: A new conceptualization. In D.A. Crighton & Towl, G.J. (Eds.). *Forensic Psychology* (3rd edition). Chichester: Wiley.

Howitt, D., & Sheldon, K. (2007). The role of cognitive distortions in paedophilic offending: Internet and contact offenders compared. *Psychology, Crime & Law, 13*(5), 469–486. doi: 10.1080/10683160601060564

Key Stage History (n.d.) The Great Fire. Retrieved from: https://www.keystagehistory.co.uk/keystage-1/the-great-fire-at-ks1/

Hurley, W., & Monahan, T. M. (1969). Arson: The criminal and the crime. *E-Journal of the British Journal of Criminology, 9*, 4–22. Retrieved from https://academic.oup.com/bjc

Jackson, H. F., Hope, S., & Glass, C. (1987). Why are arsonists not violent offenders? *International Journal of Offender Therapy and Comparative Criminology, 31*(2), 143–151. doi: 10.1177%2F0306624X8703100207

Jones, L. F. (2004). Offence paralleling behaviour (OPB) as a framework for assessment and interventions with offenders. In A. Needs & G. Towl (Eds.) *Applying Psychology to Forensic Practice*. Oxford: Blackwell/British Psychological Society.

Kane, S. (1982). Holiness ritual fire handling: Ethnographic and psychophysiological considerations. *Ethos, 10*(4), 369–384. Retrieved from http://www.jstor.org/stable/3696947

Karkanas, P., Shahack-Gross, R., Ayalon, A., Bar-Matthews, M., Barkai, R., Frumkin, A.,... Stiner, M. C. (2007). Evidence for habitual use of fire at the end of the Lower Paleolithic: site-formation processes at Qesem Cave, Israel. *Journal of Human Evolution, 53*(2), 197–212. doi:10.1016/j.jhevol.2007.04.002

Kolko, D. J., & Kazdin, A. E. (1992). The emergence and recurrence of child firesetting: A one-year prospective study. *Journal of Abnormal Child Psychology, 20*(1), 17–37. doi: 10.1007/BF00927114

Konvalinka, I., Xygalatas, D., Bulbulia, J., Schjødt, U., Jegindø, E. M., Wallot, S., ... Roepstorff, A. (2011). Synchronized arousal between performers and related spectators in a fire-walking ritual. *Proceedings of the National Academy of Sciences, 108*(20), 8514–8519. doi: 10.1073/pnas.1016955108

Koson, D. F., & Dvoskin, J. (1982). Arson: A diagnostic study. *Bulletin of the American Academy of Psychiatry and the Law, 10*(1), 39–49.

Labree, W., Nijman, H., Van Marle, H., & Rassin, E. (2010). Backgrounds and characteristics of arsonists. *International Journal of Law and Psychiatry, 33*(3), 149–153. doi: 10.1016/j.ijlp.2010.03.004

Lee, R. (2019). *An Exploration of the Experiences of Moderate Fire Users in the Community* (unpublished undergraduate dissertation). Newcastle University, Newcastle, England.

Lindberg, N., Holi, M. M., Tani, P., & Virkkunen, M. (2005). Looking for pyromania: Characteristics of a consecutive sample of Finnish male criminals with histories of recidivist fire-setting between 1973 and 1993. *BMC Psychiatry, 5*(1), 47. doi: 10.1186/1471-244X-5-47

Livesley, W. J. (2007). A framework for integrating dimensional and categorical classifications of personality disorder. *Journal of Personality Disorders, 21*(2), 199–224.

Long, C. G., Fitzgerald, K. A., & Hollin, C. R. (2015). Women firesetters admitted to secure psychiatric services: Characteristics and treatment needs. *Victims & Offenders, 10*(3), 341–353.

Lyng, S. (1990). Edgework: A social psychological analysis of voluntary risk taking. *E-Journal of the American Journal of Sociology, 95*(4), 851–886. Retrieved from https://www.jstor.org/journal/amerjsoci

Lyng, S. (2005). Introduction: Edgework and the risk-taking experience. In S. Lyng (Ed.). *Edgework: The Sociology of Risk Taking.* (pp. 3–17). New York, NY: Routledge.

Lynn, D. C. (2014). Hearth and campfire influences on arterial blood pressure: Defraying the costs of the social brain through fireside relaxation. *Evolutionary Psychology, 12*(5), 147470491401200509.

MacDonald, G., & Leary, M. R. (2005). Why does social exclusion hurt? The relationship between social and physical pain. *Psychological Bulletin, 131*(2), 202–223. doi: 10.1037/0033-2909.131.2.202

Mann, R. E., Hanson, R. K., & Thornton, D. (2010). Assessing risk for sexual recidivism: Some proposals on the nature of psychologically meaningful risk factors. *Sexual Abuse, 22*(2), 191–217.

Maruna, S. (2001). *Making Good.* Washington, DC: American Psychological Association.

Maruna, S., & Mann, R. E. (2006). A fundamental attribution error? Rethinking cognitive distortions. *Legal and Criminological Psychology, 11*(2), 155–177. doi: 10.1348/135532506X114608

Maslow, A. H., Hirsh, E., Stein, M., & Honigmann, I. (1945). A clinically derived test for measuring psychological security-insecurity. *The Journal of General Psychology, 33*(1), 21–41. doi: 10.1080/00221309.1945.10544493

McMurran, M., Fyffe, S., McCarthy, L., Duggan, C., & Latham, A. (2001). Stop & think!': Social problem-solving therapy with personality-disordered offenders. *Criminal Behaviour and Mental Health, 11*(4), 273–285. doi: 10.1002/cbm.401

Mears, D. P., Cochran, J. C., & Beaver, K. M. (2013). Self-control theory and nonlinear effects on offending. *Journal of Quantitative Criminology, 29*(3), 447–476.

Messer, W. S., & Griggs, R. A. (1989). Student belief and involvement in the paranormal and performance in introductory psychology. *Teaching of Psychology, 16*(4), 187–191. doi: 10.1207%2Fs15328023top1604_4

Mistry, J., Bilbao, B. A., & Berardi, A. (2016). Community owned solutions for fire management in tropical ecosystems: Case studies from indigenous communities of South America. *Philosophical Transactions of the Royal Society B: Biological Sciences, 371*(1696), 1–10. doi: 10.1098/rstb.2015.0174

Mistry, J., Berardi, A., Andrade, V. et al. (2005). Indigenous Fire Management in the cerrado of Brazil: The Case of the Krahô of Tocantíns. *Human Ecology, 33,* 365–386. https://doi.org/10.1007/s10745-005-4143-8

Murray, D. R., Fessler, D. M., & Lupfer, G. (2015). Young flames: The effects of childhood exposure to fire on adult attitudes. *Evolutionary Behavioral Sciences, 9*(3), 204. doi: 10.1037/ebs0000038

NASA (2017). The Sun. Retrieved from: https://www.nasa.gov/sun

Nunez, C. (2019). What are Fossil Fuels? Retrieved from: https://www.nationalgeographic.com/environment/energy/reference/fossil-fuels/

Nutt, D., King, L. A., Saulsbury, W., & Blakemore, C. (2007). Development of a rational scale to assess the harm of drugs of potential misuse. *The Lancet, 369*(9566), 1047–1053.

Ó Ciardha, C., & Gannon, T. A. (2012). The implicit theories of firesetters: A preliminary conceptualization. *Aggression and Violent Behavior, 17*(2), 122–128. doi: 10.1016/j.avb.2011.12.001

Ó Ciardha, C., Tyler, N., & Gannon, T. A. (2015a). A practical guide to assessing adult firesetters' fire-specific treatment needs using the four factor fire scales. *Psychiatry, 78*(4), 293–304. doi: 10.1080/00332747.2015.1061310

Ó Ciardha, C., Barnoux, M. F., Alleyne, E. K., Tyler, N., Mozova, K., & Gannon, T. A. (2015b). Multiple factors in the assessment of firesetters' fire interest and attitudes. *Legal and Criminological Psychology, 20*(1), 37–47. doi: 10.1111/lcrp.12065

Palmer, E. J., McGuire, J., Hounsome, J. C., Hatcher, R. M., Bilby, C. A., & Hollin, C. R. (2007). Offending behaviour programmes in the community: The effects on reconviction of three programmes with adult male offenders. *Legal and Criminological Psychology, 12*(2), 251–264. doi: 10.1348/135532506X138873

Parker, C. H. (2015). *On the Evolution of Human Fire Use* (unpublished doctoral thesis). The University of Utah, UT, USA. Retrieved from https://pdfs.semanticscholar.org/e221/0a2 5bb2f553fcdcaba39c385145debe19791.pdf

Paulhus, D. L. (1998). *Paulhus Deception Scales (PDS): The Balanced Inventory of Desirable Responding-7*. North Tonawanda, NY: Multi-Health Systems Inc.

Perrin-Wallqvist, R., & Norlander, T. (2003). Firesetting and playing with fire during childhood and adolescence: Interview studies of 18-year-old male draftees and 18–19-year-old female pupils. *Legal and Criminological Psychology, 8*(2), 151–157. doi: 10.1348/135532503322362933

Pervan, S., & Hunter, M. (2007). Cognitive distortions and social self-esteem in sexual offenders. *E-Journal of Applied Psychology in Criminal Justice, 3*(1), 75–91. Retrieved from http://www.apcj.org

Pinsonneault, I. L. (2002a). Fire safety education and skills training. In D. Kolko (Ed.). *Handbook on Firesetting in Children and Youth* (pp. 219–260). San Diego, CA: Academic Press.

Pinsonneault, I. (2002b). Developmental perspective on children and fire. In D. J. Kolko (Ed.). *Handbook of Firesetting in Children and Youth* (pp. 15–32). London: Academic Press.

Polaschek, D. L., & Gannon, T. A. (2004). The implicit theories of rapists: What convicted offenders tell us. *Sexual Abuse, 16*(4), 299–314. doi: 10.1177%2F107906320401600404

Prins, H., Tennent, G., & Trick, K. (1985). Motives for arson (fire raising). *Medicine, Science and the Law, 25*(4), 275–278

Presdee, M. (2000). *Cultural Criminology and the Carnival of Crime*. London, England: Routledge.

Presdee, M. (2005). Burning issues: Fire, carnival and crime. In M. Peelo & K. Soothill (Eds.). *Questioning Crime and Criminology* (pp. 69–82). London, England: Routledge.

Pyne, S. J. (1998). Forged in fire: History, land, and anthropogenic fire. In W. Balée (Ed.). *Advances in Historical Ecology* (pp. 62–103). New York, NY: Columbia University Press.

Pyne, S. J. (2016). Fire in the mind: Changing understandings of fire in Western civilization. *Philosophical Transactions of the Royal Society B, 371*, 2–8.. https://doi.org/10.1098/rstb.2015.0166

Pyne, S. J. (2019) *Fire: A Brief History* (2nd edition). Seattle: University of Washington Press.

Reinhard, J. R. (1941). Burning at the stake in mediaeval law and literature. *Speculum, 16*(2), 186–209. doi: 10.2307/2853611

Rice, M. E., & Harris, G. T. (1991). Firesetters admitted to a maximum security psychiatric institution: Offenders and offenses. *Journal of Interpersonal Violence, 6*(4), 461–475. doi: 10.1177%2F088626091006004005

Rice, M. E., & Harris, G. T. (1996). Predicting the recidivism of mentally disordered firesetters. *Journal of Interpersonal Violence, 11*(3), 364–375. doi: 10.1177%2F088626096011003004

Riddell, W. R. (1929). Judicial execution by burning at the stake in New York. *E-Journal of the American Bar Association Journal, 15*(6), 373–376. Retrieved from https://www.americanbar.org/groups/journal/

Ritchie, E. C., & Huff, T. G. (1999). Psychiatric aspects of arsonists. *Journal of Forensic Science, 44*(4), 733–740.

Rix, K. J. (1994). A psychiatric study of adult arsonists. *Medicine, Science and the Law, 34*(1), 21–34.

Robinson, O. C. (2014). Sampling in interview-based qualitative research: a theoretical and practical guide. *Qualitative Research in Psychology, 11*(1), 25–41. doi:10.1080/14780887.2013.801543

Rocque, M., Posick, C., & Paternoster, R. (2016). Identities through time: An exploration of identity change as a cause of desistance. *Justice Quarterly, 33*(1), 45–72. doi: doi.org/10.1080/07418825.2014.894111

Rogers, R. (2000). The uncritical acceptance of risk assessment in forensic practice. *E-Journal of Law and Human Behavior, 24*(5), 595–605. Retrieved from: https://www.apa.org/pubs/journals/lhb/

Rossano, M. J. (2007). Did meditating make us human? *Cambridge Archaeological Journal, 17*(1), 47–58.

Sandgathe, D. M. (2017). Identifying and describing pattern and process in the evolution of hominin use of fire. *Current Anthropology, 58*(S16), 360–370.

Sassenberg, K., & Ditrich, L. (2019). Research in social psychology changed between 2011 and 2016: Larger sample sizes, more self-report measures, and more online studies. *Advances in Methods and Practices in Psychological Science, 2*(2), 107–114.

Schoenstatt Scotland. (2015). Understanding why we Light a Candle in Church. Retrieved from http://www.schoenstatt.co.uk/understanding-why-we-light-candles-in-church/

Schur, E. M. (1969). *Our Criminal Society: The Social and Legal Sources of Crime in America.* Englewood Cliffs, NJ: Prentice-Hall.

Seligman, M. E., & Csikszentmihalyi, M. (2000). Positive psychology: An introduction. *American Psychological Association, 55*(1), 5–14. doi: 10.1037///0003-066X.55.1.5

Seligman, M. E., Steen, T. A., Park, N., & Peterson, C. (2005). Positive psychology progress: Empirical validation of interventions. *American Psychologist, 60*(5), 410. doi: 10.1037/0003-066X.60.5.410

Sell, A. N. (2011). The recalibrational theory and violent anger. *Aggression and Violent Behavior, 16*(5), 381–389. doi: 10.1016/j.avb.2011.04.013

Sharpe, J. A. (2005). *Remember, Remember: A Cultural History of Guy Fawkes Day.* Cambridge, MA: Harvard University Press.

Sherrell, R. (2021). *Examining the Relationship between Fire Interest and Firesetting: Contributions of Previous Experience with Fire and Self and Emotional Regulation* (master's dissertation, Open Access Victoria University of Wellington| Te Herenga Waka).

Smith, O., & Raymen, T. (2018). Deviant leisure: A criminological perspective. *Theoretical Criminology, 22*(1), 63–82.

Spencer-Oatey, H. (2004). Introduction. In H. Spencer-Oatey (Ed.) *Culturally Speaking: Managing Rapport through Talk across Cultures* (pp. 1–8). London, New York: Continuum.

Stets, J. E., & Burke, P. J. (2014). Self-esteem and identities. *Sociological Perspectives*, *57*(4), 409–433. doi: 10.1177/0731121414536141

Sykes, G. M., & Matza, D. (1957). Techniques of neutralization: A theory of delinquency. *American Sociological Review*, *22*(6), 664–670. doi: 10.2307/2089195

Taylor, J. L., Thorne, I., Robertson, A., & Avery, G. (2002). Evaluation of a group intervention for convicted arsonists with mild and borderline intellectual disabilities. *Criminal Behaviour and Mental Health*, *12*(4), 282–93. doi: 10.1002/cbm.506

Taylor, J. L., Thorne, I., & Slavkin, M. L. (2004). Treatment of fire-setting behaviour. In W. L. Lindsay, J. L. Taylor & P. Sturmey (Eds.). *Offenders with Developmental Disabilities* (pp. 221–241). West Sussex, England: John Wiley and Sons.

Taylor, J. L., Robertson, A., Thorne, I., Belshaw, T., & Watson, A. (2006). Responses of female fire-setters with mild and borderline intellectual disabilities to a group intervention. *Journal of Applied Research in Intellectual Disabilities*, *19*(2), 179–190. doi: 10.1111/j.1468-3148.2005.00260.x

Taylor, S. C., & Gassner, L. (2010). Stemming the flow: Challenges for policing adult sexual assault with regard to attrition rates and under-reporting of sexual offences. *Police Practice and Research: An International Journal*, *11*(3), 240–255. doi: 10.1080/15614260902830153

Thomson, A., Tiihonen, J., Miettunen, J., Sailas, E., Virkkunen, M., & Lindberg, N. (2015). Psychopathic traits among a consecutive sample of Finnish pretrial fire-setting offenders. *BMC psychiatry*, *15*(1), 1–8.

Topp, D. O. (1973). Fire as a symbol and as a weapon of death. *Medicine, Science and the Law*, *13*(2), 79–86. doi: 10.1177/002580247301300202

Towl, G. J. (2015). Concluding themes: Psychological perspectives and futures. In D. A. Crighton & G. J. Towl (Eds.). *Forensic Psychology.* (pp. 437–442). West Sussex, England: Wiley.

Towl, G. J. (2018). Tackling sexual violence at universities. *The Psychologist*, *31*, 36–39.

Towl, G. J., & Crighton, D. A. (1996). *The Handbook of Psychology for Forensic Practitioners*. New York, NY: Routledge.

Tyler, N., Gannon, T. A., Ó Ciardha, C., Ogloff, J. R., & Stadolnik, R. (2019). Deliberate fire-setting: an international public health issue. *The Lancet Public Health*, *4*(8), e371–e372.

Tyler, N., & Gannon, T. A. (2020, in press corrected proof). The classification of deliberate firesetting. *Aggression and Violent Behavior*, 101458. https://doi.org/10.1016/j.avb.2020.101458

Tyler, N., Gannon, T. A., Lockerbie, L., & Ó Ciardha, C. (2018). An evaluation of a specialist firesetting treatment programme for male and female mentally disordered offenders (the fip-mo). *Clinical Psychology & Psychotherapy*, *25*(3), 388–400. doi: 10.1002/cpp.2172

Tyler, N., Gannon, T. A., Dickens, G. L., & Lockerbie, L. (2015). Characteristics that predict firesetting in male and female mentally disordered offenders. *Psychology, Crime & Law*, *21*(8), 776–797.

Tyler, N., Gannon, T. A., Lockerbie, L., King, T., Dickens, G. L., & De Burca, C. (2014). A firesetting offense chain for mentally disordered offenders. *Criminal Justice and Behavior*, *41*(4), 512–530. doi: 10.1177/0093854813510911

Ullrich, S., & Coid, J. (2011). Protective factors for violence among released prisoners—Effects over time and interactions with static risk. *Journal of Consulting and Clinical Psychology*, *79*(3), 381.

Vaughn, M. G., Fu, Q., DeLisi, M., Wright, J.P., Beaver, K.M., Perron, B.E., & Howard, M.O. (2010). Prevalence and correlates of fire-setting in the United States: Results from the national epidemiological survey on alcohol and related conditions. *Comprehensive Psychiatry*, *51*(3), 217–223. doi: 10.1016/j.comppsych.2009.06.002

de Vogel, V., de Vries Robbé, M., de Ruiter, C., & Bouman, Y. H. (2011). Assessing protective factors in forensic psychiatric practice: Introducing the SAPROF. *International Journal of Forensic Mental Health, 10*(3), 171–177.

de Vries Robbé, M., Mann, R. E., Maruna, S., & Thornton, D. (2015). An exploration of protective factors supporting desistance from sexual offending. *Sexual Abuse, 27*(1), 16–33.

de Vries Robbé, M., de Vogel, V., Koster, K., & Bogaerts, S. (2015). Assessing protective factors for sexually violent offending with the SAPROF. *Sexual Abuse, 27*(1), 51–70.

Visitvalencia.com (2021). Fallas of València. Retrieved from: https://www.visitvalencia.com/en/events-valencia/festivities/the-fallas

Ward, T. (2017). Prediction and agency: The role of protective factors in correctional rehabilitation and desistance. *Aggression and Violent Behavior, 32*, 19–28. doi:10.1016/j.avb.2016.11.012

Ward, T., & Beech, A. (2006). An integrated theory of sexual offending. *Aggression and Violent Behavior, 11*(1), 44–63. doi: 10.1016/j.avb.2005.05.002

Ward, T., & Brown, M. (2004). The good lives model and conceptual issues in offender rehabilitation. *Psychology, Crime & Law, 10*(3), 243–257. doi: 10.1080/10683160410001662744

Ward, T., Hudson, S. M., Johnston, L., & Marshall, W. L. (1997). Cognitive distortions in sex offenders: An integrative review. *Clinical Psychology Review, 17*(5), 479–507. doi: 10.1016/S0272-7358(97)81034-3

Ward, T., Polaschek, D. L., & Beech, A. R. (2006). *Theories of Sexual Offending*. Chichester, England: Wiley.

Watt, B. D., & Ong, S. (2016). Current directions of risk assessment in deliberate firesetters. In R. M. Doley, G. L. Dickens & T. A. Gannon (Eds.). *The Psychology of Arson: A Practical Guide to Understanding and Managing Deliberate Firesetters.* (pp. 167–184). Oxon, England: Routledge.

Weisman, J. S., & Rodebaugh, T. L. (2018). Exposure therapy augmentation: A review and extension of techniques informed by an inhibitory learning approach. *Clinical Psychology Review, 59*, 41–51. doi:10.1016/j.cpr.2017.10.010

Whitaker, D. J., Le, B., Hanson, R. K., Baker, C. K., McMahon, P. M., Ryan, G., ... & Rice, D. D. (2008). Risk factors for the perpetration of child sexual abuse: A review and meta-analysis. *Child Abuse & Neglect, 32*(5), 529–548.

Willig, C. (2013). *Introducing Qualitative Research in Psychology*. Berkshire, England: McGraw-Hill Education.

Winder, B. (2009). Positive aspects of fire: Fire in ritual and religion. *E-Journal of the Irish Journal of Psychology, 30*(1–2), 5–19. Retrieved from https://www.tandfonline.com/loi/riri20.

Wrangham, R. W., Jones, J. H., Laden, G., Pilbeam, D., Conklin-Brittain, N., Brace, C. L., ... & Blurton Jones, N. G. (1999). The raw and the stolen: Cooking and the ecology of human origins. *Current Anthropology, 40*(5), 567–594. doi: 10.1086/300083

Wrangham, R. (2010). *How Cooking Made Us Human*. London, England: Profile Books.

Wrangham, R. (2017). Control of fire in the paleolithic: Evaluating the cooking hypothesis. *Current Anthropology, 58*(S16), S303–S313.

Wrangham, R., & Carmody, R. (2010). Human adaptation to the control of fire. *Evolutionary Anthropology: Issues, News, and Reviews, 19*(5), 187–199. doi: 10.1002/evan.20275

Wright, R. (2017). *Why Buddhism Is True*. New York: Simon & Schuster.

Wright, S. (1996). Examining what residents look for in their role models. *Academic Medicine: Journal of the Association of American Medical Colleges, 71*(3), 290–292. doi: 10.1097/00001888-199603000-00024

Yin, S. (2016). Smoke, Fire and Human Evolution. *The New York Times*. Retrieved from https://www.nytimes.com/2016/08/09/science/fire-smoke-evolution-tuberculosis.html.

Zajonc, R. B. (1968). Attitudinal effects of mere exposure. *Journal of Personality and Social Psychology, 9*(2, Pt.2), 1–27. doi.org/10.1037/h0025848

Index

Note: *Italicised* folio indicate figures, **bold** indicates tables and with "n" indicates endnotes.

'acceptable' behaviour 16–17, 35–39
"accidental" discovery of fire 9
active stages of fire use 72, **73**
adaptation to fire 9, 13
adult firesetting 3, 31–32
aftermath stages of fire use 72, **73**
Andrews, D. A. 36–37
anthropogenic fire use 8, 19n1
anthropology 4, 91, 96–97
anti-social cognition 31
application 93–94; preliminary theory of
     fire use 58–61
arson 1, 20; act of 3; crimes 40; conviction
     39, 52–53, 56, 59; criminalised fire use
     78; multi-factorial theories 2; offence
     43, 48, 66; psychological research 22–33;
     recidivistic 31; reconceptualisation of 11;
     as social problem 96
arsonists 1; characteristics of 22, 27–30;
     conviction 25–27; psychologically
     harmful effects 84; social status 56
assessment 94; forensic 63–64; generic 28;
     idiosyncratic approach 27; pre-trial
     psychiatric 32; and rehabilitation 3;
     risk 26, 33, 59, 63, 65, 67, 73
assessment of people who set fires
     63–76; dynamic considerations 68–71;
     forensic assessment 63–64; offence
     analysis 71–73; precipitating factors
     71–73; predisposing factors 64–67;
     risk monitoring and management 73–75

Bachelard, G. 20
Barnoux, M. F. 32
Barrowcliffe, E. R. 24, 29
BDSM (Bondage and Discipline, Sadism and
     Masochism) 97
Beech, A. 58, 61
Beech, A. R. 43
Bengkulu Malay 12, 17, 69
Berdychevsky, L. 96
Birch, L. L. 69, 87
Blakemore, C. 36
'bonfire night' 16, 75
Bonta, J. 36–37
Botoeva, G. 36
Breaching of religious and moral
     norms 36
Brett, A. 2, 25
Bullis, M. 17
Burke, P. J. 49
Burning Man Festival 15
Butler, H. 80

Canter, D. 66–67, 94
carnival of crime 37
caveats 22–25, 89
Centre of Research and Education in
     Forensic Psychology (CORE-FP) 3–4
change in messaging 86–89, **88**
Chief Fire Officers Association (CFOA) 86
cognitive behavioural therapy 81
cognitive distortions 56, 74

continuum of fire use (CoFU) 39–42, *40*, 44; conceptualisation 65, 78; treatment and intervention with people who set fires 78–79

Continuum of Fire Use Theory (CoFUT) 45–53, *46*, 59–60, 79–85, 92, 98; conviction 74; human-fire relationship 62; preliminary theory 43; security 56

CORE-FP *see* Centre of Research and Education in Forensic Psychology

COVID-19 37

Criminal Damage Act 1971 36

criminalised fire use 16–17, 22, 35, 38–41, 44, 52, 54, 58, 71, 78–80, 92, 96

Criminal Justice System (CJS) 23, 34

culture and fire use 85–86

Danforth, L. 15

dangerousness: of people who light fires 33; recidivism and 25–27

Darwin, Charles 7

Daykin, A. 23

deductive approach 30

Dickens, G. L. 27, 31

Ducat, L. 26, 29

Dvoskin, J. 25

dynamic behaviour model 2, 31

edgework 52, 80

Edwards, M. J. 3, 26

emotionally expressive/need for recognition 31

England: Regulatory Reform (Fire Safety) Order of 2005 20; Smoke and Carbon Monoxide Alarm Regulations of 2015 20

exposure therapy (ET) 81

external consistency 58, 61–62

external recognition 51, 62

Faulk, M. 27

Fawkes, Guy 16

fertility/heuristic value 59

Fessler, Daniel 1, 8–10, 12, 16–17, 54, 69, 85, 93, 95

Fineman, K. R. 31

FIP-MO *see* firesetter intervention programme for mentally disordered offenders 3, 77, 80–82, 85, 90

FIPP *see* firesetter intervention programme for prisoners

fire 6–19; "accidental" discovery of 9; adaptation to 9, 13; in celebrations 15–16; control of 2, 8; discovery of 7–13;

for entertainment 15–16; fire play 6, 9, 12–19, 40, 59, 69, 83, 95; interest 25, 29, 31, 67–69, 82, 97; lighting 71; messaging **88**, 88–89; misuse of 4; production of 8; psychological aspects of 13–15; role in evolution of species 6, 10; and sense of self 71; setting 45; as tool for indigenous peoples 12

fire and rescue services (FRSs) 3, 20, 86–87, 95

firefighters 2

fire-related behaviour 2, 4, 16, 34–35, 40, 79, 93, 95

fire-related beliefs 18, 68–70

fire safety: awareness 28; education 4, 58, 86–87, 95; in England 20; officers 17; promotion 58

firesetter intervention programme for prisoners (FIPP) 3, 77, 80–82, 85, 90, 94

firesetters 4; characteristics of 22, 27–30, 32; dichotomy 24–25; quantitative research 24; treatment needs 68

firesetting: adult 3, 31; challenges 2–3; convictions 39, 81; defined 1; institutional 44, 48, 53; needs 29; prevalence 24; prevention 4, 9, 78; progress 3–5; psychological research 22–33; treatment 13–14

fire-specific constructs 28

fire use 2, 4, 35–42; Continuum of Fire Use (CoFU) 39–42, *40*; criminalised 38–39; culture and 85–86; dichotomy 35–38; history 64–67; holistic conceptualisation of 92–93; non-criminalised 38–39; process questions 73; *see also* preliminary theory of fire use

Fire Use Matrix (FUM) 67, 97

Fisher, J. O. 69, 87

Flahavin, Mary 40

"forbidden" nature of fire 17

forensic assessment 63–64; *see also* assessment

forensic psychology 78, 92, 95, 98; *see also* positive psychology

forensic status 23–24

Foster, J. E. 40, 89, 95

Fritzon, K. 23, 66–67, 94

FRSs *see* fire and rescue services

functional analysis model 31

functional use 12, 44, 65

Gallagher-Duffy, J. 29
Gannon, T. A. 17, 23–24, 28, 39, 69–70, 80–81, 85
Gayton, W. F. 13
gender 22–23
generalist and specialist hypothesis 28
Global North 11–13, 66
"good fires and bad fires" 40
Good Lives Model 84
Good Lives Model (GLM) 41, 56, 81, 84
Goudsblom, J. 11, 15
Gowlett, J. A. 8, 12
Grace, R. C. 3, 26
Great Britain 11–14, 16–18, 20, 35–39, 42, 56, 66, 70, 85–87, 95, 97
grievance 31
Grounded Theory (GT) 44

Hall, J. R. 16
Hamilton, L. 23
Harris, G. T. 25, 28
Heyman, J. M. 36
"hidden fire" 12; *see also* fire
Higgins, E. T. 48
Hope, J. 38
Horsley, F. K. 22, 44, 61
Hudson, S. M. 59
human-fire relationship 4, 7, 11, 19, 34, 42, 45–46, 62, 65, 93
Hurley, W. 25

identity 23, 49–50, 53, 57, 71, 82–84
idiosyncratic approach 27, 32–34
ignition stages of fire use 72, **73**
immediacy nature 47
immediate gratification 46–48
implicit theories (ITs) 32, 34n1
inductive approach 30
instigation stages of fire use 72, **73**
'intervention programmes' 3, 77–78, 86, 90, 94–95

Jackson, H. F. 9, 31, 81

Kane, S. 15
Kazdin, A. E. 17
King, L. A. 36
Kolko, D. J. 17
Konvalinka, I. 15
Koson, D. F. 25

Lee, R. 61
legal acts 36

Lexical Decision Task (LDT) 29
lighting a fire 58, 71–72; *see also* fire
Lindberg, N. 29
Lupfer, G. 12
Lyng, S. 52
Lynn, D. C. 13

Malamuth, N. 96
Maruna, S. 57
mechanisms of defence 56
mediator 46, 48–49
messaging, change in 86–89, **88**
Miller, S. 23
Mistry, J. 12, 16–17
misuse of fire 4, 20–34; arson and firesetting 22–33; implications 33–34; risk 33
Monahan, T. M. 25
motivation 2, 12, 16, 30, 32, 57, 66–67, 72
multi-faceted human-fire relationship 11, 31, 43
multi-factor theories 30–32
multi-trajectory theory of adult firesetting (M-TTAF) 30–32, 70, 92
Murray, D. R. 70, 86, 97

narrative repair 57
natural selection 10–11, 19, 47
neutralisation 56
non-criminalised fire use 35, 38–39
non-firesetters 4, 21, 24–25, 29, 34, 67–68, 92, 98
'non-firesetting' 17, 21–22, 38–39
Norlander, T. 17, 24
Nutt, D. 36–37

Ó Ciardha, C. 68, 70–71, 82, 85, 94
offence analysis 71–73
offence chain theories 32–33
offence paralleling behaviour (OPB) 74
'one size fits all' approach 2–3, 63, 68, 75

Parker, C. H. 8–9
Perrin-Wallqvist, R. 17, 24
Pinsonneault, I. L. 14, 17–18
planning stages of fire use 72, **73**
Polaschek, D. L. 43
positive psychology 41–42, 64–65, 92; *see also* forensic assessment
predominantly criminalised fire users 44
preliminary theory of fire use 43–62; application 58–61; evaluation 61–62; methodology 43–45; psychological wellbeing 53–58; *see also* fire use

Presdee, M. 4, 13, 15, 37–38
psychological behaviour 36
psychological wellbeing 53–58, 83–85
psychology 4; forensic 78, 92, 95, 98; positive
    41–42, 64–65, 92
Pyne, S. J. 8–9, 11, 14–15

recidivism: dangerousness and 22, 25–27;
    research 26
reckless fire play 45, 65
recreational use 44, 65; see also fire use
redemptive narratives 57
Regulatory Reform (Fire Safety) Order of
    2005 (England) 20
religious use 45, 65
Rice, M. E. 25, 28
risk assessment 2, 26, 33, 59, 63, 65, 67, 73;
    see also assessment
risk factors 26–27, 31, 33, 65
risk monitoring and management 73–75
Risk of Sexual Violence Protocol (RSVP) 41
risk paralleling behaviour 74–75

Sandgathe, D. M. 8, 95
Saulsbury, W. 36
Schur, E. M. 37
security 53, 54–56, 83–84
self-esteem 51–53
self-preservation 56–58, 74
sense of self 49–53, 71, 82–83
sensory stimulation 59, 70, 72
setting fire 24, 27–28, 35, 38–39, 45, 65, 78
Sherrell, R. 12, 86, 98

Simonsen, B. 17
social construction of fire 93
sociology 4, 91, 96–97
Spencer-Oatey, H. 6
spiritual and ritualistic use 45, 65
Stets, J. E. 49
Sugarman, P. A. 31
symbolism and fire 13–15; see also fire

theoretical perspectives 30–33
Topp, D. O. 14
transient emotional state 46–49, 80–82
transitory nature 47
treatment and intervention 94–95
treatment and intervention with people
    who set fires 77–90; early intervention
    85–89; psychological wellbeing 83–85
Tyler, N. 32, 39
typologies 30–32

'unacceptable' behaviour 16, 35–38
University of Kent 3

Vaughn, M. G. 24
vocational use 45, 65

Ward, T. 43, 58, 61
Winder, B. 13–15, 54, 93
Wrangham, R. W. 8–11
Wright, R. 47

Yardley, L. 62
Yin, S. 56

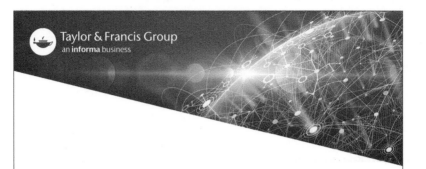

For Product Safety Concerns and Information please contact our
EU representative GPSR@taylorandfrancis.com Taylor & Francis
Verlag GmbH, Kaufingerstraße 24, 80331 München, Germany